NATIONAL INSTITUTE SOCIAL SERVICES LIBRARY
NO. 42

# OLD AGE HOMES

*Housing*

# National Institute Social Services Library

# Old Age Homes

## ROGER CLOUGH
*Lecturer in Social Work, University of Bristol*

London
**GEORGE ALLEN & UNWIN**
Boston          Sydney

First published in 1981

GEORGE ALLEN & UNWIN LTD
40 Museum Street, London WC1A 1LU

**British Library Cataloguing in Publication Data**

Clough, Roger
    Old age homes. – (National Institute social
services library; no. 42)
    1. Old age homes – England
    I. Title    II. Series

ISBN 0–04–362043–4
ISBN 0–04–362044–2 Pbk

Set in 10 on 11 point Times by Grove Graphics, Tring
and printed in Great Britain
by Richard Clay (The Chaucer Press) Ltd,
Bungay, Suffolk

# CONTENTS

*To my Mother and my Father*

# FOREWORD

In this disturbing and compassionate book Roger Clough describes the day-to-day life of men and women, residents and staff who live and work at The Pines, an old age home.

He shows the double bind in which residents and staff are enmeshed: a bind created when the prevailing belief that elderly people should keep active is combined with a wish on the part of staff to care for residents and a desire in most old people to be looked after at least to some extent. In demonstrating this situation Roger Clough blames neither staff, residents, nor relatives. All are caught in the confusion in society about the process of ageing and suitable provision for the elderly.

It is appropriate that Roger Clough undertook the participative research for this book when he held a fellowship from the Central Council for Education and Training for Social Work, and that at the time of publication he is a lecturer in a university social work department, because his book demonstrates the value and the possibilities of a social work approach. He shows what an accepting and non-judgemental attitude means in action. He attempts to understand but never to blame and he does not do this from a position of uncertainty or unconcern about what is right for elderly people. That he knows, but he knows too the problems of achieving it.

The book is also a demonstration of the application of the social sciences to the lives of real people and will offer an example to students who find it hard to know the meaning of integrating theory and practice, something which they are exhorted to achieve. They will also learn how to combine feeling and ideas in a way which enriches understanding.

Roger Clough's book is important for its content but also for the way it is written. It illustrates the welding of care and thought which typifies good social work, whether it be research writing, teaching, or practice.

PHYLLIDA PARSLOE
*Professor of Social Work,*
*University of Bristol*

# ACKNOWLEDGEMENTS

———◆———

As a residential practitioner I worked in approved schools with young people (today's community homes with education). My interest in residential work with the elderly developed during several years as a lecturer to students, primarily from old people's homes, on a residential social work course at Bristol Polytechnic. At intervals I would be asked what I really knew or understood about old people's homes. And I asked myself what were the similarities and differences between residential work with children and the elderly.

The fellowship awarded to me by the Central Council for Education and Training in Social Work gave me a practical opportunity to examine these questions.

I am grateful to the Council for this opportunity and to those in the Department of Social Services in Somerset who agreed to my working in one of the county's homes, in particular to Larry Pritchard and John Fellowes.

Peter Righton provided me with stimulating supervision during the study period, as did colleagues at Bristol Polytechnic. More recently, when working on this book I have received valuable support, comment and detailed criticism of the text from Christopher Beedell, Roger Bullock, Roy Parker, Phyllida Parsloe and Michael Power at Bristol University. Margaret Windsor has typed both my study notes and the numerous drafts of this book. Phrases like 'residential home' have been written so often that now they type themselves!

Above all my thanks go to the staff and residents of The Pines whom I got to know so well for the way they allowed me to share in their lives. For me, often prone to forget people's names, the vividness with which I can recall not only names but faces, features, expressions and incidents is a testimony to all that my stay at The Pines meant to me.

# OLD AGE HOMES

# INTRODUCTION

◆

Two residents of an old people's home, The Pines, describe a typical day.

MISS BRINTON: After breakfast we sit in the lounge and read, have coffee. It's a long period between dinner and tea. When I think of how I used to gallop around! I look forward to visitors, get to know other people's visitors. Bingo seems useless. Here I come up to bed at eight. At home about nine with a milky drink in bed. It takes a long time to get undressed and change the bag [a colostomy bag], one hour or more. I like to do things for myself. I was used to having help with bathing. Here it's more convenient and I'm not embarrassed. At home I had my bath at a regular time from an attendant. Here I have one on the first day and one the last Saturday [she was in for a holiday]. I'm glad to have a bath when it's convenient for the staff but I liked the choice. I'm not rushed – make sure I have long enough – I know I can't do it by myself.

MR MURPHY: It's difficult to get dressed – annoying not being able to tie laces, I don't like having to ask. I usually get up, shave and wash, an 'up and downer'. Get up about five past seven (used to be earlier at home), use a wet razor. I can't see well but it's OK, move off at ten past and down to breakfast at twenty-five past eight. I enjoy the meals, they're good and well cooked – but they give you too much. They can't cook it how you would like it. Usually go up to the sitting room and read the paper. Sleep for half an hour, read the paper, then coffee at eleven. I might move around; go up and down the passage and walk round the place, in the summer I'd go round the garden.

Sit down and talk in my sitting room, never been in other sitting rooms. I know most of them, stop as I go past to talk. The difference isn't the home, the difference is me, can't see well, sight is my biggest loss, gradual loss – had three operations. Came like a yellow blur in the middle of the eye – they operated – and it was worse.

After lunch, sleep, walk, talk, TV and tea. Then TV again, I stay up until about ten, sometimes nearly eleven. I get a bit bored in the morning before eleven. Read the paper and then now't to do. I could go for a walk but I would be in the way of the cleaners.

Twice a year I go to the British Legion stunt [a party] – I've got two tickets now but I can't get in touch with my daughter, I trust her, she's my eyes. They could phone for me. Don't suppose it would be difficult to get anyone to write – I'm not much of a one for asking favours of anyone. When you've lived so long you're used to doing everything for yourself – think twice about asking. Sometimes go to bingo. I like the slide shows and concerts they have.

This book is based on a detailed study of this particular old age home. It illustrates events and records the feelings, such as those above, of residents, staff, relatives and other professional groups – doctors, nurses, health visitors and social workers. Based on this evidence some explanations are suggested for various patterns of events and some conclusions are drawn about practice in old age homes.

Old age alters people's pictures of themselves and of life. Two comments from the extracts above illustrate this: 'When I think of how I used to gallop around', and 'The difference isn't the home, the difference is me'. Each individual is faced with a different set of difficulties and dilemmas, so there is no single answer to the question 'What is the secret of a happy or successful old age?'. Nor can a residential home hope to put right crippling physical or emotional handicaps. What it should be able to do is to provide a place where an individual's needs are met in a way that allows her the maximum control of her life.

The first four chapters place such accounts as this in the context of a wider discussion about residential homes and ageing, together with a brief discussion of the methods used in this study. From there the bulk of the book, Chapters 5 to 9, provide the flesh – detailed consideration of admission and departure, of significant events for staff and residents, together with a longer study of two residents. The last four chapters begin the task of considering the relevance of this material to more general issues – processes of control, ageing in institutions and the objectives of residential establishments.

There are parts of the material that show sadness, harshness and insensitivity. They are included here not to attack old age homes but from beliefs that such homes are needed, that they can be good places to live in and that a clearer understanding of processes that take place within them is essential.

Finally there are some stylistic points. First, the names of the home and the residents have been altered, though the identity of the residents is maintained. Secondly, since the majority of those in old age homes (staff and residents) are women, I have used feminine pronouns (she, her) rather than the clumsy he/she. It is more difficult to find an adequate title for the place where residents live. 'Old people's home' is the most widely used, though some people refer to 'homes for the elderly' in a belief that the phrase sounds better. 'Home' tells us nothing about the size of the establishment and carries expectations of 'homeliness' which are unrealistic. 'Institution' has overtones of regimentation but may be used in a technical sense to describe an organisation and the building which houses it. Both words – home and institution – will be used in this study to avoid excessive repetition, together with words like centre and establishment. The problem of terminology is more fully discussed elsewhere (Clough 1979a and b).

# Chapter 1

---

## OLD AGE HOMES – MYTHS AND REALITIES

Living in an old age home evokes pictures of apathy, dependence and sadness. This is not the image most of us have about our own life in old age. Attitudes seem crystallised in that of Sir Keith Joseph (1972), addressing a one-day conference on residential work, when he looked down from the platform at a group of staff from old age institutions: 'Your old people would rather not be in residential homes, wouldn't they?' he said. Such assumptions, based on the negative aspects of residential homes in general and of old age establishments in particular, have led to policy statements about the desirability of enabling the elderly to stay in their own homes. In this chapter these assumptions are examined and questioned.

### ATTITUDES TO AGEING

The starting point is a consideration of attitudes to ageing. Many of the fears that surround old age establishments are in reality fears about old age itself. Old age homes confront us with conspicuous evidence of problems that *may* come with ageing – problems such as confusion, senility, severe and multiple handicap, and the resultant dependence on others. Ten individuals may live in their separate homes sitting for hours doing nothing. If those ten people are grouped together and all seen sitting for hours doing nothing, the image is more than ten times as powerful. No wonder a district nurse responded to a questionnaire by writing:

> The whole aspect of living in an old people's home fills me with horror. The patients appear to me like lodgers in a silent hotel, a place with no pulse, fed, slept and sheltered. Armchairs in rooms, round the edge of the wall, just sitting. The sad thing about the whole thing is that patients sit there from choice . . . I feel they look so pathetic just sitting in silence in armchairs.

Old age is bearable in prospect as long as we can maintain a picture of contentment and continued interest in the world around, and as long as physical or mental impairment does not hit too hard. It is difficult to maintain a picture of successful ageing when some or all of these factors do not apply. The old age home presents society with the apathy or handicap of residents *en masse*. It is easy to forget that old age anywhere may be as unpleasant. Similarly by focusing on the poverty of the life of some residents it is easy to put aside our anxieties about our own old age.

Anxiety about old age has two important aspects: physical deterioration which may affect body or mind; and purposelessness resulting from loss of role, death of friends or relatives, poverty and isolation. Both aspects, physical deterioration or purposelessness, may occur inside or outside a residential home.

To ignore this is to fall into the trap of distorting the reality of old age. An American writer, Gubrium (1973), calls this process 'The myth of the golden years'. A part of this myth concerns the social context of old age. One view of this social context 'is that of the alleged well-being of old people who continue to maintain their own neighbourhood household . . . The first of these images . . . conceives of a self-sufficient couple in an older neighbourhood of homes, who maintain a mutually satisfactory round of daily life. Both are portrayed as actively involved in a variety of crafts and hobby-like activities. Both maintain active local connections in neighbourhoods that are "just as I remember them".'

Gubrium continues, 'Not only are social contexts considered felicitous but so are the relationships between old people as well as their activity. Four images of interaction and activity should be noted: (1) the idea of growing old together; (2) the indulgent intergenerational portrayal of the aged; (3) the ideal active "busyness" of the elderly; and (4) the simple advice of planning for retirement.'

Gubrium explodes the myth – many old people are not in their own neighbourhoods or surrounded by a network of relationships. They may have been rehoused, living in lodgings or flats. The myth ignores the movement of neighbours and the crime rate that leaves the old too frightened to leave their homes. Finally, many old are single, do not get on well with their children and do not have the resources of money or health to remain 'busy' in old age.

It will be apparent later that most professional workers, when considering their own old age in response to questionnaires, thought in terms of the freedom old age would bring and greater opportunities to pursue interests. This is a very important side of old age, rightly stressed by organisations for the aged. But the other side of the coin is weariness and bitterness.

A part of Gubrium's attack is directed against what has been termed the *activity theory* of ageing. This theory, associated particularly with

Havighurst (see Havighurst and Albrecht, 1953), proposes that old people age successfully if society accepts the value of the old and ascribes them publicly valued roles. In particular old people should substitute new activities in old age for those which they give up on retirement. An offshoot of this idea is the claim that people need to plan for old age, which has led to the development of pre-retirement classes to encourage such planning.

Gubrium criticises activity theory on the grounds that activity is seen mostly in terms of work-like situations that are active and visible, and stereotypically middle class. The quality of social relationships is ignored. In addition the high degree of physical dependence and the limited roles available to old people are not examined. It became apparent that some people with high morale had low activity.

An alternative understanding of needs in old age was introduced by Cumming and Henry (1961). They suggested, in what has been termed the *disengagement theory*, that society withdraws from the older person. The individual co-operates in a process of disengagement between himself and society. This is a mutual process. Happiness in old age depends on the individual and society accepting this role for the elderly. While disengagement theory takes into account the needs of society for younger, more active people to replace the older, it may ignore the needs of the elderly. In particular it assumes that this process must take place for all societies and all individuals within that society.

A more recent theme in research work into ageing has been to consider the basis on which one can assess life satisfaction in old age. Havighurst (1968) shows how emphasis has shifted away from the either/or debate surrounding the conflict between the activity and disengagement theories. Citing the Kansas City Study of Adult Life he states (p. 304):

The results of this study indicated that neither the activity nor the disengagement theory was adequate to account for the observed facts. While there was a decrease of engagement in the common social roles related to increasing age, some of the people who remained active and engaged showed a high degree of satisfaction. On the whole those who were most active at the older ages were happier, but there were many exceptions to this rule.

This study carried on the work of others in looking for a personality dimension as a factor that influenced successful ageing. An analysis was produced which was based on three dimensions – personality, role activity and life satisfaction. Havighurst concludes (p. 308):

Of the three dimensions on which we have data – activity, satisfaction and personality – personality seems to be the pivotal dimension in describing patterns of ageing and in predicting relationships between level of activity and life satisfaction.

In contrast Gubrium, in his socio-environmental approach, emphasises the interplay of two factors – activity resources and activity norms. Activity resources are those resources which enable a person to do the things she wishes. They include money, housing, local facilities, social support and health. Activity norms are the norms that an individual has come to accept and share in common with others about what she should be doing.

This theory stresses the importance to old people of expectations about activity. The old will be satisfied when they are able to do what they and others regard as appropriate. Mr Murphy (p. 1 above) found his health worse – he was nearly blind and could move only with difficulty. Yet he did not like having to ask other people to tie his shoe laces. So his resources did not match his norms. Gubrium argues that someone may be said to be coping or have high morale when her resources match the norms set by herself and others. The theory is particularly helpful in explaining why many residents at The Pines found it hard to adjust to their worsening physical state.

Thus attitudes to old age institutions are influenced by fears about old age itself. In addition there is no agreement about what constitutes or results in successful old age. The old may not have the resources to match expectations and, while it is possible to envisage providing the old with more money or better facilities, it is unlikely that much can be done about deterioration in health. Consequently it is necessary to adjust norms as well as to look for better resources.

## ATTITUDES TO RESIDENTIAL LIVING

Old age homes have similarities to organisations like homes for the physically handicapped or long-stay hospitals in which residents are expected to be permanent. Yet all such organisations, along with most other residential establishments, are regarded as second best to living in one's own home. There are only a few exceptions. In situations where there is a high degree of voluntary entry to establishments (i.e. there are several other living styles available and the residential home is the preferred choice) or where great importance is attached to the purpose for entry (e.g. boarding school) residential living is seen more favourably. Religious establishments, hotels, communes and boarding schools come into this category. Social service type institutions – for children, the mentally or physically ill, the mentally or physically handicapped, the old – fall into the second-best category. The negative aspects of such establishments have been well documented and have become part of the conventional wisdom. Residential institutions have been criticised for almost as long as they have been in existence. Criticism has been intense since the 1950s. Bowlby (1951) cited the dangers for children in institutions from maternal deprivation. Barton (1959) stated that living in institutions could produce a set of problems (which he called institutional neurosis) more difficult to eradicate than the original reason for admission. Goffman, in a series of major essays brought together in *Asylums* (1961), discussed the totality and pervasiveness of institutional regimes. The more total the regime, the more an institution devised rituals to ensure that physical constraints (such as walls and locked doors) were matched by social pressures to conformity and he illustrated this theme by examining the 'stripping' of the person that took place at admission.

With this as background has followed a succession of studies of types of institution – for example, Townsend (1962) on old people's homes, Morris and Morris (1963) on Pentonville, Morris (1969) on subnormality hospitals, Meacher (1972) about homes for the elderly confused. These have added their weight to the criticism of residential institutions.

## ATTITUDES TO OLD AGE HOMES

Today's elderly have vivid memories of the workhouse, the predecessor of local authority old people's homes. The workhouse has become a symbol of harsh, unimaginative and regimented living. Whether such a picture is true or not, the tradition lives on. The old consider entering a residential home to be a sign of failure and, on admission, expect to be compliant.

Townsend's study was a significant landmark in the development of attitudes to old age homes. After the Second World War there were hopes that new and smaller residential homes would lead to more satisfactory living conditions for the elderly. Townsend showed the inadequacy of building programmes but also the inadequacy of life-style within many purpose-built establishments. The view of the old age home as second best was reinforced.

The Williams Committee (1967), set up to examine the training needs of staff in residential homes and acknowledge the importance and the skill of the work, expressed similar sentiments:

One basic fact has to be kept in mind, that even the best residential home is likely to be ranked as second best in the mind of those who come into it. It cannot replace the independence a person enjoys in his own home or give what an affectionate family can provide. Everything is different from what he has been accustomed to for so long. The rooms may be warm and bright and prettily decorated, the chairs comfortable, the food good and plentiful. But they are different and take getting used to. And one's new companions are not those whom one has known all one's life, who understand the names that crop up in the conversation or recognise the references to past experiences. It is a sad thing not only to suffer the infirmities of old age but to find oneself among strangers at a time of life when it is difficult to make new friends.

Not surprisingly there have been demands to put resources into 'community' and 'preventive' work, though I have argued elsewhere that this contrast between 'residential home' and 'community' is inaccurate and unhelpful, for residential establishments are very much part of the community (see Clough, 1978a).

Townsend (1962) suggests

a number of far-reaching proposals . . . to reduce progressively the number of communal homes (in the first instance by closing the former workhouses) and to replace them in part by sheltered housing and in part by a slight extension of the hospital system . . . to enlarge greatly the domiciliary services, mainly by creating a local authority family help service, and to develop general practitioner group practices.

Meacher (1969) argues for a similar change of policy:

The Government should declare an unequivocal commitment to reverse the emphasis of social policy in old age from care in institutions to care in the wider community. This should be based not only on considerations of cost-effectiveness or on the well documented pathologies of institutional life, but on the urgent need to give priority to developing preventive services and to keeping the individual within the therapeutic framework of the family circle and the surrounding network of friends and neighbours, with its interchange of services between generations.

So the stereotype became established that people, whether young or old, mentally ill or subnormal, were better off in their own homes. Residential institutions have been regarded as evils, whether necessary or unnecessary evils.

'Of course there are some exceptions; but in the main the conditions of our residential institutions are appalling.' This statement from a *Guardian* editorial (27 January 1978) typifies this attitude, as does a report by Conrad Jamieson for Cheshire Social Services in 1973:

On the surface an old age home might seem to be only a geriatric ward in disguise. The picture it presents is all too often one of dependency, discouragement, confusion and the regressive and senile behaviour of second childhood. Yet below the surface is an unrealised potential for the institutionalised old to live normal, healthy and self-sufficient lives. Why isn't this potential being better realised even in well run and modern homes . . . ?

The symptoms of senility which proliferate in old age homes cannot be put down as due solely to the ageing process, but must be attributed largely to the institution of the old age home itself in creating what we call 'situational senility' which is induced by a particular set of environmental factors. The harsh truth would seem to be that residents of old age homes do not grow senile in spite of institutionalisation but because of it. Two factors in particular would seem to explain situational senility:

(a) the forcibleness of the uprooting the old person undergoes in entering a home
(b) the role expectations within the home itself which covertly or overtly encourage dependent and regressive behaviour.

In the *Guardian* was the comment on this report: 'even the most modern home schemes offer little hope of mitigating the effects of institutionalisation to any appreciable degree. The resident often enters a home in a demoralised state, feeling rejected by family or friends with whom it will be difficult to maintain relationships'.

The potential dangers are magnified by an awareness of the high degree of dependence of residents and the possibility of maladministration and cruelty by those running the home. Numerous examples could be given of inefficiency and cruelty in a range of residential establishments. In old age homes one illustration of violence was the conviction of a superintendent for assaults on residents. Witnesses stated:

The residents sat in the same chairs, they were not allowed to do anything for themselves. They were like robots.

[His] attitude to patients made them subdued and crestfallen.

The superintendent pinned a resident in his chair against the table and yanked back his head and pushed food into his mouth, at the same time shouting at him. This was an unpardonable and unlawful use of force [the prosecution claimed].

Mr (M) would not always move his legs. [His] reaction was to kick him on the legs to make him walk. One mealtime he fell on the floor. As he lay there on the floor [he] kicked him on the top of his legs. (Extracts from *Oxford Mail*, 1973)

Any suggestion that residential care could be beneficial has, by comparison, been slight. Discussion of such benefits as have been mentioned has been primarily in relation to treatment-oriented units, especially with young people. But Harris (1968) states that a large majority of the residents of old age homes enjoy living in the home. Simpson (1971) examines the implications of the different regimes of three old age homes and concludes that one style of living is preferable because it produces mobile, physically active and social residents. Most recently Brearley (1977), though accepting that the best residential home will be second best in the mind of the individual, stresses that 'work with the elderly can be interesting, worthwhile and successful'.

### DOMICILIARY OR RESIDENTIAL CARE

Righton (1977) makes a similar point.

> Catalogues of the disadvantages of residential care are all too common: often compiled by academic psychologists and sociologists whose experience of communal living is remarkable chiefly for its brevity, they are usually referred to collectively in articles and lecture halls as the 'literature of dysfunction'. Lists of advantages, by contrast, are as rare as air on the top of Mount Everest, and about as invigorating.

There is no doubt of the potential dangers in residential care but there are potential dangers in families and in living! There is too often a facile assumption that domiciliary services are by nature superior. In the same way anything that can claim to be 'preventive' may enhance its legitimation. If the dangers and also the cost inherent in residential care are put in the background, an important question can emerge. Are cruelty and regimentation inevitable factors of residential living or are they examples of bad practice? Put the other way this becomes – is there anything intrinsic about residential homes to suggest that living in a well-run residential home is not as adequate as living in a well-run home in the wider community?

There are fallacies in the belief that for *all* people, at *all* times, living in the wider community is preferable. This stereotype is supported by a number of assumptions. The first of these places an idealised model of domiciliary care alongside a picture of inadequate residential care.

The strengths of domiciliary care – the maintenance of an established pattern of life, the 'normality' of living – are seen in ideal terms. This means that the inherent possibilities domiciliary services could provide for some are assumed to be available, functional and appropriate to all. This is contrasted with 'the well-known pathologies of residential life' (Meacher, 1969), in other words the problems inherent in residential living – loss of freedom to make decisions, loss of independence, loss of one's own home, isolation. In fact the existing model is contrasted with the ideal and the conclusion that the ideal is best is not surprising.

It would be as easy to do the reverse procedure. One could discuss residential homes in ideal terms – as being therapeutic communities that enable the elderly to lead fuller lives – and contrast this with the squalor, the deprivation, the apathy, the lack of relationships and the failure of domiciliary services outside them. Such a study could show that meals on wheels are too rushed, too infrequent and often thrown away; that social workers, health visitors and doctors have been 'unable to spot and ensure treatment of the miseries of old age' (Goldberg, 1970); that visits by volunteers are irregular and patronising; that in spite of the mobilisation of considerable resources many old people remain lonely, friendless and isolated. Either method of idealising one type of provision and comparing this with an existing service is mistaken.

Another assumption is that 'home is always best'. The belief in the superiority of home life seems based on the fact that it is the norm. But this does not mean that this ought to be the accepted pattern for everybody. Indeed, we may well be moving into an age when the isolation of the family is rejected more often in favour of communal living. Living on one's own is not necessarily better than living with other people.

A very real danger of present research is that it accepts the present norms and attempts to provide substitutes for them. Thus we attempt to substitute 'residential care' for 'home life' and we assess the adequacy of residential care by the degree to which it approaches the norm of home life. The basic assumptions themselves need questioning – in this case that home is always best – and in particular one has to examine whether an individual has ever lived according to the norm.

Of course, home is the best for some people. Just because that statement is so obviously true one must be on one's guard against presuming it is true for everybody. Many old people may never find real warmth, real nurture and care and real friendship while living in their own homes. This may be so whatever quantity, quality and type of domiciliary services are offered, for it is doubtful if such services can ever supply such needs. Some old people may be loved and cherished in the setting of a residential home in a way that is not possible in any other type of care. The very 'residentialness', to use a clumsy word, which involves physical caring and the supplying of emotional needs is obviously applicable only to the residential home.

Of course, physical needs can be met in such a way that emotional needs are not fulfilled. Food can be served so sloppily that it is clear that the cook has no interest in the person for whom the food is provided; but equally presentation of food can demonstrate the warmth of the caring relationship. So living in a residential unit may supply the needs of some old people.

There are other strengths to residential work which could be singled out – twenty-four-hour observation and care, an ability to deal with the rapid change in feeling on top of the world or under the weather that old people face, a greater likelihood of lending support in the many aspects of loss that have to be faced, a chance for the resident to do more because some of the problems of living are removed, the probability that the miseries of old age will be better cared for.

It is important in this context to realise that many of the old people at present in residential care are those who have been unable to sustain a normal pattern of relationships at home. So it is unreasonable to judge the residential unit solely by the degree to which normal relationships appear to exist.

Another aspect of this discussion is cost-effectiveness. Residents in old age institutions are becoming older and more dependent at admission. Their needs are considerable and to meet such needs adequately via domiciliary services would necessitate a vast growth in such services. Domiciliary provision for the highly dependent is only cheaper while it is less adequate – while it fails to provide twenty-four-hour cover, laundry services, regular meals, help with bathing, toileting, housework, cooking. The list could be immense (Hobman, 1977).

## THE INTERTWINING OF TWO MYTHS

The two myths –the myth of the golden years and the myth of the evil institution – when intertwined appear to present an irrefutable argument that the old are best kept out of unpleasant residential homes to live an active and fulfilled life from their own home base. Limits and provisos must be placed on such a statement.

The prevailing attitude, that stresses the limitations or even harmful effects of residential care, is sustained by many who are not in a situation where they have to make a choice about living arrangements in old age. It may well be that, with family around and strong neighbourhood ties, a residential home seems abhorrent; is it so abhorrent when one is old and lonely with many friends already dead? Indeed, how many people making the sort of statements that are made about inadequate residential care are faced with the emotional deprivation of cooking or cleaning only for oneself after having done this for a family?

Another aspect of the 'golden years myth' is the esteem given to independence. It seems widely accepted that one of the virtues of domiciliary care is that it encourages old people to do things for themselves and the principle is becoming accepted for residential care as well. Of course, independence and self-help are important goals. But they should not be over-riding goals. The morality of encouraging some old people to go on struggling through most of their waking day to do little other than maintain themselves and the fabric of their environment should be questioned. Outsiders, even families, may believe it is right to persuade the old to carry on in their own homes. Mrs Richardson (p. 65 below) describes how the household tasks had got too much and she was relieved to be cared for, even though she was now farther from her family.

Peter Townsend (1962) lists nine fundamental principles which might be embodied in 'a realistic and enlightened general policy for the aged'. His fourth principle is that an individual should be helped 'to live as independently as possible in a home of his own'. His commitment to the value of domiciliary care means that the *potential* of the residential home is ignored. Two further sentences highlight this: 'On the available evidence we are obliged to conclude reluctantly that the residential home, at least as it has taken shape in the post-war years, is misconceived and inappropriate. It does not fit rationally into a coherent system of services for the elderly and handicapped.' While it is important to examine the significance of Townsend's survey of what life was like for residents of old people's homes, it is not necessary to adopt the conclusion that resources should be shifted to domiciliary services.

The problem for old age homes is compounded because of uncertainty about their purpose. Should they be the 'hotels for pensioners' of Aneurin Bevan's dreams or are they better seen as special housing provision? In addition there is far less clarity about normal patterns of caring for the old than about child-rearing. Adults have lived through childhood; adults are usually available to rear children and the norms of such rearing would command wide acceptance. By contrast those planning provision for the old have not been old themselves; families may not be available to provide care, and the old, with adult responsibility for choice of life-style that is not given to children, will present a greater scatter of views (Clough, 1978b).

Townsend uses his analysis of the shortcomings of residential institutions to propose major changes in provision. By contrast Goldberg (1970), while illustrating the failures of social workers, spells out the implications of her research for the task of the field worker. It is similarly possible to consider the shortcomings of residential work *and* the implications for the task to be performed. Until this is done the quality of work with the elderly will be the poorer.

Homes for the elderly are in existence; demand for them is increasing faster than provision. These residential homes will remain in existence for the forseeable future. Whether or not they are ideal living situations, they are necessary ones. Constant denial of the value of their task will lead to a further lowering of the morale of staff. As a first step to improving morale and consequently the life-style and happiness of those within the homes it is essential that a clearer understanding be developed of the processes in an old age home.

Margaret Tilley (1971) suggests that happiness is the main objective of a residential home and that the home which promotes this is indeed a therapeutic community. She continues: 'It is worth noting that in work with the aged one can be an uninhibited hedonist, for, unlike children, their characters are made or marred and one does not have to take into account character formation.'

Earlier in her paper she writes: 'Perhaps more than anything, at this present stage of development in residential provision for the elderly, we need some imaginative and exploratory thinking so that we can ask the right questions about old people's needs and wishes as a necessary preliminary to discovering how these can best be met.'

This study is an attempt to ask the right questions about old people's needs. It shows daily happenings within one home and offers explanations for some of these events. Where there is dissatisfaction with the life-style that is portrayed, whether dissatisfaction of reader or author, such feeling may be a spur to finding more appropriate ways of meeting the needs of the elderly within a residential home.

# Chapter 2

---

# STYLES OF OLD AGE HOMES

There are so many assumptions about the elderly that it is essential to be able to place them in a context. The typology of old age homes that is introduced (p. 22 below) allows events to be examined in relation to specified variables. Such a framework is valuable but must not lead to oversimplification. One of the major goals of social research should be to avoid simplistic explanations (see pp. 18–19 below). In the first part of this chapter I give the rationale for the framework developed later.

## ATTITUDES TO AGEING: 'IT'S FOR THEIR GOOD'

One of the aspects of residential homes that I find disturbing is the ease with which it is possible for staff, especially senior staff, to translate their attitudes into action. One matron explained to me that her residents were given margarine rather than butter because it was better for their health; another served an afternoon cup of tea only to those able to walk to the dining room because activity was good for them. It is by this most seductive phrase that the lives of many old people are ruled. The old, in and out of residential homes, are advised to drink more or to drink less, to keep active, to get out, to get up and to eat up because *it is good for them*. So the whims and fancies of staff are readily translated into action. I was anxious to find out what were the beliefs of the staff and residents about the appropriate styles of living. How far could such attitudes be linked to particular assumptions about the ageing process?

The uncertainties as to what constitutes successful ageing have already been mentioned. They are of particular importance here. In caring for children, adults draw on their own experience of being a child; in caring for the old there is no first-hand experience. No wonder some old people insisted staff did not know 'what it is like to be old'. Comments from residents such as 'They'll understand when they are old that old people must not be rushed' were frequent.

STYLES OF OLD AGE HOMES

In addition there is less written about the needs of the old than those of children. In residential child care part of the task is to provide the resources for healthy development in the light of knowledge available about children's needs. This is an aspect of what Beedell (1970) calls 'parenting'. He states that parenting involves 'holding', 'nurturing' and 'provision for the development and maintenance of personal integrity'. There is no word to describe the task of 'parenting your elders' but, even were such a word available, there is little analysis of what the components of that task should be. For example, Beedell states about nurturing: 'All societies have arrangements for encouraging, and sometimes insisting on the development of skills; social, physical and intellectual.' Such a global statement could not be made about nurturing the elderly.

It is, of course, arguable that residential care of the elderly should take as its prime task the holding aspect of provision. 'All societies have customs and rituals designed to ensure the dependent child's survival and to protect him from danger, discomfort and distress. In doing so they give the child mainly good experiences of care, comfort and control' (Beedell, 1970). Yet, while 'holding' is an essential aspect of the task of caring for the old, it should not become the only one. The elderly have nurturing and development needs also. The body of knowledge of what constitutes such needs is minimal. Consequently individual assumptions are likely to play a larger part in meeting such needs.

## A BROAD EXPLANATION OF EVENTS

It is at this stage that it is necessary to repeat the statement that old age institutions are an integral part of the community. Many studies have examined residential institutions as separate entities. Morris (1969), by contrast, makes the point: 'However much it may appear so from the inside, subnormality hospitals are not islands unto themselves, but are a part of a wider community.' Attitudes of staff and residents are not formed in isolation. Consequently it was decided for this study to include an assessment of the attitudes of people outside the institution – in this case field social workers, doctors, health visitors, district nurses and relatives of residents.

So one part of the picture presented here is drawn around attitudes to ageing. Another part shows attitudes to residential living. If residential homes are regarded as second best and less than adequate, in particular if entry to a residential home is regarded as failure, then it would not be surprising to discover that residents found the life dissatisfying. This fact has been demonstrated in other situations. Miller and Gwynne (1972) argue in relation to homes for the disabled that residents may be 'socially dead' before admission. The inability to fulfil roles such as breadwinner and husband is itself a sign of failure. Entry to a residential home only confirms an existing situation. Tobin and Lieberman (1976) show how acknowledgement that one is going to enter into a residential home is a key factor in apathy within a residential home. In other words entry to a residential institution confirms the perception of oneself as an individual without valid social roles. Passivity and dependence comes from the process that *precedes* admission as well as that which takes place after entry to a home. An example from my own study illustrates this (Clough, 1978c):

> Mrs Smith had lived in a sheltered housing scheme prior to admission to an old people's home. She described to me her life, entertaining the family, and her involvement in a wide range of activities. She was a lively member of a local church, baked more cakes for the coffee morning than anyone else and had a positive picture of her past. Within the residential home her life had changed – physically, since bouts of arthritis left her crippled and in severe pain on occasion; spiritually, since she could no longer believe in a God who had allowed so much to happen to her; socially, for she had cut off links with her church and past friends. She did retain close links with her family and, though she described herself as bitter, kept going at some things such as knitting . . .
>
> The temptation is to consider that these situations arise from the ill effects of institutional living. The dreaded institutionalisation has struck again! Such an explanation is far too simple. It presumes that the ill effects arise from institutional life, whereas there may be other significant factors.
>
> Mrs Smith's life prior to admission to a residential home was very full. Her life after admission was not. It is in such situations that institutionalisation is so seductive an explanation. However, her change in attitude and life-style is much better explained by the anticipation of living in a home. She was clear that living in a residential home was a visible indication of one's reduced purpose in society. Her response to this was to initiate the severing of past ties. It was her assumptions about the status of residents in old age homes that led to her bitterness. *The actual life-style within the home was not the reason for her change in attitude.*

A second example illustrates the way that the feeling of rejection by one's family plays a significant part in life within the institution (Clough, 1978c).

> By contrast, Mrs Draxton appeared to have given up. Her moaning and complaints were constant – she was bored but felt there was nothing else to do. She sat and sat; residents and staff tried to arouse

her interest but gave up, discouraged. Again, this was a contrast to her former life, struggling to educate her daughter as a doctor, taking pride in her ability at crafts. Her daughter, with whom she had been living, was going to move away; the daughter thought her mother would be better off in a residential home. Mrs Draxton was still bemused when I met her, months after admission, as to why she needed to be in a home and how she had got there. She was facing loss and a major break in the continuity of her life.

## THE FUNCTIONS OF RESIDENTIAL ESTABLISHMENTS

One of the ways in which I tried to draw some of these threads together was to consider different approaches to running old age homes.

Goffman (1961), in his study of total institutions, listed five categories:

(1) institutions established to care for persons felt to be incapable and harmless; these are the homes for the blind, the aged, the orphaned and the indigent;
(2) institutions for those who are incapable but comprise an unintended threat to society;
(3) institutions for the protection of society from intended danger;
(4) institutions for the transmission of work-like skills;
(5) institutions for those wishing to retreat from society.

Moss (1975) has a different set of functions:

healing;
compensation for deprivation or disablement;
acquisition of certain common social skills/habits;
the facilitation of certain work or the acquisition of special roles or skills;
the acquisition of caste/class/party values and habits;
deterrence or punishment;
protection of the community from 'harmful' influences;
protection of inmates from corruption, exploitation;
elimination or neutralisation of inmates.

Meacher (1972) discusses more specifically the functions of separatism in social policy. He reviews a wide range of institutions and considers to whom the benefits of such separatism accrue. Such segregation, he argues, needs to be understood in terms of the interests of the beneficiaries of dissociation. For example, the remainder of society benefits from prisons, rich and powerful families from public schools. He continues:

Since then segregation is by nature manipulative, however in-
directly, it follows that, except where it is exercised voluntarily and
the beneficiaries of dissociation are identical to those to whom it is
applied, its consequences are likely to be at best limiting and at
worst punitive.

Meacher uses this as a basis for examining special residential homes
for the confused elderly. There are similar important questions about
the functions of other old age institutions. Who profits from such
establishments, what types of selection and restriction exist, in what
ways does segregation take place?

Old age institutions do not fit readily into any of Moss's categories
though they may be thought of as providing compensation for deprivation, or healing. They are mentioned specifically in the first of
Goffman's groupings: 'institutions caring for persons felt to be incapable and harmless'. On the sort of analysis used by Meacher it is
possible to suggest that they benefit relatives and younger able-bodied
people, that restrictions are in terms of indefinite residential living
because no other alternative is possible.

The functions of the old age home are significant, for greater clarity
is needed about the tasks it carries out. In addition it is apparent that
it is easier to assess whether some functions are satisfactorily fulfilled
than others. There is a variety of ways of assessing whether schools
have transmitted instrumental skills successfully, of which the most
obvious is to assess examination results. Similarly it is possible to see
whether prisons can contain prisoners without escapes, whether isolation
hospitals prevent the spread of disease; even when considering establishments such as community homes and special schools, when goals
are less certain, it is possible to look at factors such as integration with
family and community, academic achievements, social achievements,
ability to 'survive' without recourse to welfare establishments.

Indeed, much recent writing has stressed measurement, whether of
behaviour ratings of children in the Measure of Treatment Potential
or the linking of staff–child interaction with performance in tests of
reading and arithmetic in units for autistic children (Grygier, Bartak
and Rutter, 1975). In this way it is possible to discover which regime
will lead to an increase in the achievement of the child.

Without the end measurement (in this example the performance
tests) it is less easy to use any scales that may be devised. It is the lack
of measurable objectives that make long-term caring institutions for
adults difficult to assess.

Far more account has to be taken of the extent to which the
individual resident is satisfied with his current life-style and the service
provided. Though there may be severe financial limitations it may be
possible to demonstrate that one regime produces more satisfied resi-

dents than another; alternatively it may be possible to show that particular regimes produce particular results and then to allow a moral decision about which regime and result is preferred.

Pincus (1968) devised a framework for studying the institutional environment. He developed a questionnaire which was designed to provide information on four dimensions: (1) public–private; (2) structured–unstructured; (3) resource sparse–resource rich; (4) isolated–integrated.

The theme of assessment of residential homes is taken up in two recent publications, Peace, Hall and Hamblin (1979) and Hughes and Wilkin (1980). The first group of authors look for a 'quality of life' rating which draws on the experience of consumers. The second publication, while accepting 'quality of life' as a useful scale, points out the limitations of such an approach, particularly if it relies too heavily on a group of consumers who are likely to be uncritical.

Probably it is better to search for the components of 'quality of life' rather than to attempt a composite score. This will allow comparison between establishments on a range of variables, as would Pincus's questionnaire, but would not presume that there is certainty about how to score any characteristic. For example, it is useful to know that residents in one home spend more time sitting in a lounge than in another. But it must be remembered that any individual may wish to spend more or less time in the lounge. There is no right amount of public living.

## MODELS IN RESIDENTIAL INSTITUTIONS

Essentially the move to identify models in residential institutions has developed from a wish to identify characteristics and so to chart different styles of home, with implications about the impact on residents and staff. It is perhaps part of a movement that has looked for variations other than the extent to which an institution is more or less total.

So Miller and Gwynne (1972) hypothesise three models – warehousing, horticultural and organisational – in homes for physically handicapped adults. The first is linked to 'the humanitarian defence' in which 'humanitarian values apply pressure to postpone physical death for as long as possible' though the unhappiness of those whose life is prolonged may be unacknowledged. The horticultural is linked to 'the liberal defence' – 'the abnormality of the inmates is denied: it is claimed that they are 'really normal . . . by treating such a person as normal the abnormality, with its limitations, is denied.' The third model is based on a belief that the task of the organisation is to support the individual in the choice he has made about life-style. 'He may choose dependence, he may choose hyperactivity; he may modify his choice as his physical condition changes.' Whichever he chooses, the task of the organisation is to support that choice.

This approach is a base for that of Meacher (1972), who posits four models based on different philosophies: (1) euthanasia; (2) warehousing; (3) horticulture; (4) social deprivation. Only the fourth needs any elaboration. This is based on his tenet that since part of 'the causation of mental confusion among the aged entails a strong social component', then compensation should be a major factor to encourage full integration and normalisation.

Millham, Bullock and Cherrett (1975a) and Moss (1975) provide two other examples. Millham and colleagues in a study of approved schools suggest different styles of school – nautical school, senior training school, junior training school, family group school, campus school therapeutic community. They proceed to illustrate the differences in type of philosophy, organisation, systems of control and other factors.

Moss (1975) builds, perhaps, on the work of King, Raynes and Tizard (1971) who have suggested that medical and child care outlooks lead to different life-styles for institutions. Moss lists three main models – child care, educational, medical/nursing – while a fourth model, housing, ought to but does not exist in any numbers. He lists a variety of factors such as size and siting of unit, type of staff and children, and compares the differences with these three models.

### TYPOLOGY OF OLD AGE INSTITUTIONS

However, work on old people's homes has, by comparison, been minimal and heavily dependent on a survey of institutions for old people by Townsend (1962). Part of the reason for this present study was to consider what may be important variables in different lifestyles for old people in institutions.

Table 2.1   *Typology of Old Age Institutions*

| | Model of Ageing | | |
|---|---|---|---|
| CONTROL OF LIFE-STYLE BY RESIDENT | Activity | Disengagement | Socio-environmental |
| Minimal control by resident | (1) Nursing home | (4) Institution | (7) 'Home' |
| Some control | (2) Therapeutic unit | (5) Hotel | (8) Hostel |
| Maximum feasible control | (3) Retirement community | (6) Flatlets | (9) Supportive unit |

The typology I have used (Table 2.1) is developed from two variables: (1) the extent to which a resident controls her life-style; (2) different models of ageing. Its value is in the extent to which it makes *explicit* some of the assumptions which are often hidden. The names are chosen to indicate a style of life within an institution. Thus the table allows comparison between a 'nursing home' style and a 'hotel' style of institution, but I am not suggesting that all nursing homes or all hotels conform to these styles.

The models in the table illustrate some of the patterns of living that various combinations of these two variables may produce. Such models are devised as ways of describing regimes more precisely and allow for individual choice as to the most appropriate style of living.

The models are discussed in detail below. The following factors were used to compare institutions: (1) type of admission (the degree of control by the resident and others); (2) theories and assumptions about ageing; (3) aims of organisations; (4) staffing implications (staff–resident ratio, authority structures, use of uniforms, job demarcation); (5) building implications (block or units, types of lounges); (6) control systems (regulations, formal and informal expectations); (7) control of life-style by resident (indicators used – money, cleaning, daily programme, bathing, medicines and drugs, meals, furniture and decorating). The same outline is used subsequently for the study of the particular home in this study, The Pines. The details below are hypothetical outlines.

There are limitations to this approach. The precision that such an analysis may suggest cannot be wholly upheld. Institutions may fit broadly into one of these categories but the large numbers of personnel involved (staff, residents, outsiders) will not all have the same assumptions about the ageing process. Indeed, that is one of the major problems for residents who may have different assumptions from those of staff. The 'model of ageing' variable is used to indicate the predominant attitude within the institution, which is likely to be that of the staff. There are further limitations to the use of these theories. In particular a key part of the disengagement theory is that the process of disengagement involves co-operation between the individual and society. So 'disengagement' is used here to indicate a predominant attitude that the process of withdrawal from active roles is the key to successful ageing. The way in which such a view may be imposed on others is a separate, though important, question. This would relate to life inside or outside a residential establishment and is discussed by Lowenthal and Boler (1965), though not in relation to residential institutions.

Brief synopses of all nine styles of old age institutions are given below, while four styles (the nursing home, therapeutic unit, institution and supportive unit) are developed in greater detail.

The first three types are based on an activity theory of ageing. This postulates that successful ageing involves finding replacement activities for those that are given up through retirement or ill-health.

## (1) *Nursing home*

This is a staff-dominated establishment with prevailing beliefs that limbs need to be exercised; that people need to be taken out of themselves, that residents, if left alone, will become apathetic.

Many residents will have been transferred from hospital; residents are thought to need residential care because they are not fit enough to manage outside. 'They will keep you going and keep you young' residents will be told.

Stress is placed on the efficiency of the unit and on planning activities rather than the happiness or satisfaction of the residents.

A hierarchical system exists with the head known as 'Matron'; staff are nurse trained and wear uniforms; there is clear job demarcation. The building is large, necessitating much communal activity, and there are few single rooms.

Staff and residents are aware of strict rules. They are enforced by physical constraints, for example, removal of cigarettes, forced feeding, manhandling to bath, control of places of seating and sleeping, threat of transfer.

Residents have minimal control over their life-style. Pension books are held centrally. Residents are given money rarely; it is spent for them. There is great emphasis on cleaning and hygiene, with thorough cleaning of rooms every day; the more active residents are given tasks. Stress is placed on routines, and residents are expected to conform; they must join in with activities arranged for them; activities are valued because they keep people occupied. There is a fixed bath rota with close supervision by staff. All residents have the same doctor; staff call the doctor when they think necessary; staff keep and distribute all drugs. Meals are held at set times; residents must attend, must eat something and have no choice; the feeble or unwilling may be forcibly fed. Rooms are seen as belonging to the organisation; residents have no say in their decor, and few possessions around; staff enter rooms without knocking and will put away items they do not wish to have around; furniture and floor coverings may be plastic or vinyl for easy cleaning.

## (2) *Therapeutic unit*

To an activity theory is added belief in therapy and rehabilitation. Staff are dominant, but provide for resident participation. Common statements are: 'you don't have to but I'd like you to join in'; 'it's good for you'; 'if you just sit, you'll lose the ability to walk'.

Developmental aspects are stressed, as with the horticultural model.

A blind eye is turned to disabilities and so success is judged in terms of accomplishments while in reality dependence may be increasing. The resident is consulted about admission and the opportunities are emphasised.

Creativity or personal fulfilment are important (though they may be unattainable to many) alongside tasks which residents are able to manage. Less emphasis is placed on the efficiency of the organisation.

There is consultation by senior staff with junior staff and residents; the head is 'head of home' and social work trained; staff do not wear uniforms and there is an overlap of jobs. Units are smaller, perhaps wing-type, with wings radiating from a central administrative block.

There is much greater use of normative control – the expectations of staff and other residents.

Residents are encouraged to be independent and to try to perform tasks, and the attempt is seen as valuable in itself; they are encouraged also to understand money, sort out change and go out to shop, though money may be given out centrally. Baths must take place regularly, but residents are stimulated to develop skills to bath themselves; similarly with cleaning arrangements. Staff encourage residents to participate in a 'treatment programme'. There is a choice of doctor, drugs are reduced and residents may hold drugs if staff agree. Residents influence menu and meal-times, but are encouraged to 'eat up'. They are given some choice of colour schemes and bring some furniture.

### (3) *Retirement Community*

Common in America, unusual in Britain, the home offers a vision of a new life. Life continues to be active and purposeful while the resident makes decisions.

The old person decides to apply for admission. She plays a major role in appointing staff, with the consequence that the head is known as 'the manager'. Staff may wear uniforms, and have specialised jobs; they are seen more as employees. The buildings have good communal facilities including a bar, library and games rooms and residents have single rooms.

The next three types are based on disengagement theories.

### (4) *Institution*

The essential elements here are withdrawal by residents from social activities, and minimal control of life-style. Indeed the withdrawal is involuntary, being forced on the resident by practices that exist within the institution. So the resident is prevented from participating in the life of the home and is given no responsibilities for her own life-style. Regimentation and block-treatment are combined with a staff belief that it is no longer appropriate for the resident to share in the hustle of life.

Some people may be formally admitted, decisions will be made by others and the resident told that 'it will be nice to let others cook/ clean, and so on', or 'it's time you gave up'. Doctors will be influential in this process.

There is a hierarchical system with the head known as 'warden'; staff are nurse trained and wear uniforms. As with the warehouse model, staff focus on the task to be accomplished rather than the needs of the resident. Buildings will reflect the wish to observe and control residents.

There are similarities with the 'nursing home' style in terms of minimal control by residents. The basic distinction is that in this model activity is seen as something that confuses. Residents do best when they are left in a settled routine; anything out of the ordinary will be detrimental. The apathy that accompanies this style is regarded as natural: 'it's sad for them but they have to accept that their useful life is over'.

## (5) *Hotel*

The philosophy – that disengagement is natural – is similar to that above. However, residents are seen as people with influence. They must be consulted and their wishes taken account of. Residents and staff agree that a quiet life is best.

The resident is consulted about admission and encouraged because 'you will be free of all the chores'.

Staff influence over life-style remains great because staff control the resources. This is a particularly powerful situation when residents accept that they have few needs – relatives will be given their pension, and residents will be anxious to appear as gentle old people who fit in with all that is asked.

## (6) *Flatlets*

This style reflects separate living-space for the old, but within that space a contented and happy existence. Restrictions and changes in life-style have been accepted and the resident has found a satisfactory *modus vivendi*. At admission, chosen by the resident, the resident acknowledges that former roles of parent, worker, club member have much less significance; therefore she will be happier in a situation where less is expected of her.

The final three models develop from a socio-environmental theory of ageing.

## (7) *Home*

The word 'home' of the title is intended to convey the picture of the institution that endeavours 'to be just like home'. Here staff control is linked to a theory that allows differential explanation for individual residents. Staff acknowledge that individuals have different resources but they set the expectations for the group and for each resident. So one person may be expected to do more: 'what sort of life is that for someone who is as fit as she is?'. While another may be excused inactivity: 'well she's 93, you can't expect much'.

## (8) *Hostel*

In this style staff set the rules of the establishment but within that framework residents are given freedom to select their own life-styles. So staff might say: 'we ask them what they want and fit in where we can'. When consulted about admission, prospective residents will be told: 'provided you fit in with the home, you'll be able to do what you want'.

## (9) *Supportive unit*

Here resident dominance is combined with a socio-environmental theory of ageing. People are limited by resources and norms and how well they cope is dependent on how well resources and norms match. A major distinction from other styles of resident dominance is that residents may be physically dependent while making decisions about life-style.

Admission is requested by the resident who was aware that she would have greater choice of life-style in the old age home than in her own home. She would also be aware that staff would support her in her choice.

Residents play a major part in establishing the pattern of living; contracts making formal demands on staff may be drawn up. The weakness of the residents' position is that they may be a less cohesive group. But they have potential power to hire and dismiss staff. The head of the unit is known as 'the manager'; units may well be smaller, having a mixture of trained staff. It may be that fewer staff are employed or staff may change some of their functions.

The living style is controlled by the resident – with similar bounds to those that exist outside the home. Consideration must be given to fire risks and health hazards from neglect or incorrect medication. Otherwise residents are free to allow rooms to get dirty; to allow themselves to get dirty; they call the doctor when they wish; they have some choice of food, meal-times and they (or relatives) may cook some meals. Privacy is ensured by locks to doors. Residents are free to request staff help with tasks.

It is important to stress that the models are developed as a first stage in considering the link between events and attitudes and in opening up a discussion about the appropriate style for an old age establishment. Provisos need to be made in addition about the control of life-style variable.

'Control of life-style' is significant for several reasons. There is a long history to the feelings that residential institutions make people powerless. While it is necessary to consider rights for children, it is still more important that adults be given the maximum opportunity for making decisions. Studies of services for children which have used scales to measure attributes such as block treatment (King, Raynes and Tizard, 1971) have as a baseline that individual control of space or possessions is important.

King, Raynes and Tizard developed a scale – the Child Management Scale – which is designed to give a picture of the extent to which a unit is institutionally oriented or child-oriented. They pick out four areas – rigidity of routine, 'block-treatment', depersonalisation and social distance – and use questions related to these areas to give a total picture of an establishment.

'Rigidity of routine' is described as follows – 'Management practices are institutionally-orientated when they are inflexible from one day to the next, and from one inmate to another . . . ' – and includes as the first two questions:

(1) Do the children aged 5 years and over get up at the same time at week-ends as they do during the week?
(2) Do the children aged 5 years and over go to bed at the same time at week-ends as they do during the week?

In old age homes it is far more difficult at present to be sure of the components of good care. While there can be little justification for treating all of the residents in the same way, any particular resident of an old age home may choose an inflexible pattern of living and profit from going to bed and getting up at the same time.

'Block-treatment' refers to dealing with residents in batches, depersonalisation to providing no opportunities for personal possessions or privacy; both of these components provide useful ingredients for institutional analysis. However, 'social distance' again brings in a dilemma. 'Management practices are institutionally-orientated when there is a sharp separation between the staff and inmate worlds. This may be because separate areas of accommodation are kept for the exclusive use of staff, or because interaction between staff and children is limited to formal, and functionally specific, activities.' In an old age home social distance may be almost a basic human right, for residents may not wish to have intrusions made on their lives.

If it is accepted that maximum feasible control of life-style is a valid goal with the elderly it is important not to measure its attainment solely in terms of indicators which have prejudged what is the appropriate life-style. Therefore an incident, such as getting up or bathing at a regular time, may be an indication of either an inflexible regime which imposes this on a resident or an indication of a choice made by a resident and supported by the staff. The linking of 'control of life-style' and 'models of ageing' (which draws on attitudes and assumptions) allows a more appropriate examination of these issues.

The discussion of key factors in analysis of old age institutions will be picked up again in chapter 11 together with an examination of the distortion that can be created by measuring certain factors (such as control of life-style) and ignoring others (such as stability of staff and tenderness).

# Chapter 3

## PARTICIPANT OBSERVATION IN OLD AGE HOMES

On one occasion at The Pines Mrs Draxton said to a care assistant: 'I don't love you any more.' There followed some discussion amongst other residents before the care assistant replied: 'I know what that's about – she had left some things out on her bed and we put them away for her, for her own good. Well Matron wouldn't have liked it.' Mrs Draxton retorted: 'Well, I'll know for the next ten years.'

Such an episode raises basic questions about research methods and interpretation. How reliable is the evidence? Did the observer affect the outcome? Would the same result be repeated in other comparable situations? What hypotheses explain this particular event? Which is the most likely of these explanations?

This book draws on material from a study of a single establishment. The dangers in such an approach have been documented by Tizard, Sinclair and Clarke (1975). They stress the need to look at factors that make one establishment different from another:

> [Our] approach highlights the differences which exist between the institutions at the same time as it makes it possible to evaluate their effects. By contrast, early research relied heavily on the single case study, so that it could only be generalised on the untested assumption that any one institution is an adequate representative of its fellows. This book tests that assumption and shows it to be false.

Thus it would be entirely inappropriate to draw on Mrs Draxton's interaction and to presume that there was a rift between all residents and staff at The Pines, and still more inaccurate to extend the conclusion to a general assumption that in old people's homes staff and residents fail to understand each other. However, in a situation where there is little idea of what are the right questions (or the key variables) the single episode may provide useful clues.

In fact, what is offered is a series of scenarios, or photographs, of a particular home. Provided that we remember the limitations of the photograph – a particular lens was used, the photo was taken from a particular angle, in a particular light, and so on – it is a useful way of capturing some aspects of an event. Similarly with this material – some pictures of a scene are presented but the limitations must not be forgotten. Hall *et al.* (1975) also consider that, given safeguards, the case study has value. In particular they suggest that it is 'a valuable means of conveying the immensity of the task confronting those who embark upon the journey from description to generalization in this terrain'. They add that such studies are 'suited to the "action" approach and to the exploration of the meanings actors attach to their behaviour in policy-making situations'.

PLANNING AND METHODS

Following detailed study of one establishment I hoped to gain some understanding of significant events and processes. Particular aspects were specified before going into the home – attitudes to ageing, admission processes and consequent changes in life-style, the formal and informal expectations of all involved in the home, a picture of daily life, choice and control, life satisfaction objectives of the home.

*Attitude to ageing* was one of the variables used to construct the typology of old age homes. Its significance is apparent from the way actions are influenced by beliefs or assumptions. For example, one resident, Mrs Hendon, stated that the home was a hotel and that she was there temporarily.

> I go out to work for a spinning company – well I don't go now, I'm out of work, getting on for 80. Sometimes I get miserable. Now I have got the house to myself I am well occupied, I don't get bored. I've always been one for getting up early; my daughter gets up between seven and eight. I have what I fancy for breakfast. If my husband has days off we go out to dinner.

Staff members assuming either that confused old people should be humoured or that they should be confronted with reality would treat Mrs Hendon differently. Questions about 'attitude to ageing' placed some of these assumptions in a broader framework. I asked: 'What is your picture of successful ageing? What sorts of things should old people do? Is it important to keep working? Do you look forward to or dread old age? A central aspect of the study was that the assumptions of different groups were examined: these included residents, staff, relatives and workers from the neighbourhood.

The second variable, *control of life-style*, differs from the more usual analytic idea of 'institutional control'. The distinction is necessary for two reasons. First, 'control of life-style' examines the situation from the point of view of the resident and charts the extent to which a resident has mastery of her own life. Secondly, since there is little known as to which situations are found to be most restricting by the old, it is necessary to start from a study of the types of control that can be exerted by residents. In addition ideas about institutional control have developed from work with children, and it is more essential for adults in residential homes to make their own decisions since they have done so for most of their lives. Mrs Williams said that sitting and waiting for a meal made her feel like a child at school. Whether it is right or wrong, children are more used to being managed in groups than are adults. When adults find themselves in comparable situations they recall their childhood dependency.

I selected some particular moments or happenings and used these as 'indicators' of life-style. These are listed below, together with some questions.

(1) *Money* Who holds pension books? What words are used to describe the pension (e.g., 'pocket money')? If given out by staff, where is it distributed (at office, in lounges, individual rooms)? Is money spent by staff on goods they decide are necessary? Who controls expenditure of group money such as 'comfort funds' or sums raised at special events?

(2) *Cleaning* Who decides the frequency, the time and the way in which the room is cleaned? Are residents allowed to leave the room in a muddle or dirty?

(3) *Daily programme* What choice do the residents have about the time when they get up or go to bed? Are events arranged for them? Are they expected to attend various functions including occupational therapy, communion? Do residents or others initiate visits, outings? Are residents and visitors free to come and go when they wish?

(4) *Bathing* Do staff or residents decide the frequency and the time of day for a bath? Do residents have any say in the way they are bathed? (Is it possible to choose between being left to lie in a bath on one's own for a few minutes or, if worried, having constant attendance?) Do any residents bath themselves? Do residents or staff select the clothes residents wear after their bath? Who decides which staff member will bath a resident?

(5) *Drugs and doctors* Do any residents hold their own drugs? How are drugs distributed? Is there any indication of over-medication, especially of confused or awkward residents? May residents choose their own doctors? Are residents seen in private by the doctor? Are the residents able to call a doctor or is this negotiated with staff?

(6) *Meals* Is there any choice of menu? Is there any flexibility in the time of meals? Are residents allowed to miss meals if they are in

the home? How are meals served? Are there serving dishes on each table or are meals served centrally? Are residents able to negotiate what they want? Is there any pressure to eat up or not to waste? Are residents allowed to cook anything? Are residents allowed to make drinks of tea or coffee for themselves or their visitors? Is there any choice as to where a resident may sit?

(7) *Individuals' rooms*   Are residents allowed to decorate their rooms (paint the door, wallpaper or paint walls)? May pictures or ornaments be hung? What sort of furniture, if any, may be brought in? Are residents allowed to carpet their rooms? Do residents have a key to (*a*) the door, (*b*) a cupboard, or (*c*) a drawer in their room? May they put their name on the door? Is there a letterbox on the door? Are small possessions and ornaments allowed to be displayed or is it considered that they get in the way of cleaning?

The aspects for study listed earlier (p. 31) provide information which may be used to relate 'the various elements of the formal structures and processes of institutions to the informal life which operates within them' (Lambert, Bullock and Millham, 1970). However, the subsequent work of these authors at the Dartington Research Unit stresses also that their perspective tries 'to consider the dynamic implications of the individual's definition of his situation' (Millham, Bullock and Cherrett, 1975b).

So, for example, the interaction of Mrs Draxton and the care assistant cannot be understood by examining the goals of the establishment and the methods of social control. Mrs Draxton does not 'simply respond to social pressures in the manner of some robot', she evaluates her interaction with others and redefines her own position. For her this was often confusing and she felt she had a low position in the eyes of others.

*Life satisfaction tests*
There is no easy way of measuring happiness or someone's satisfaction with her life. In an interview a resident, Mrs Roberts, talked about life at The Pines.

It's a bit early to get up. My breath's bad in the morning. I do a bit, make the bed, wash, do some washing up. At nine-thirty I read the paper, look forward to that. I'd rather do without breakfast. Then some knitting, crochet and organising the football pontoon. All the days seem long. We used to get a young fellow with an electric organ, now he doesn't come. They used to enjoy it, have a sing-song. We need a public phone, we use the phone in the office. There used to be a phone in a booth in one of the lounges, it was in the wrong place, needs to be near the doors. I look forward to going to the

pub. The food is very good here but there's no choice, you can't
expect it, and they do change the menu. I sleep after lunch. I've
got my own TV but don't get a good reception. I need an outdoor
aerial. I've asked about it but I don't know what to do else. The
lounge is too hot, I'd use my room more if the TV picture was
better. Can't always watch what I want in the sitting room, I like
sport. In the summer I go outside, in the winter stay in and watch
TV. They're afraid of a mouthful of fresh air here.

How satisfied does she appear to be with her life? What extra information would a test provide?

Since 1949 there have been a variety of tests and scales developed
to examine morale or life satisfaction. These have focused on the
attitude that the individual holds towards herself and, as Gubrium
points out, this is a significant determinant of a person's control of
her own behaviour. Gubrium, in fact, sees morale as being dependent
on a match between expectations being made of an individual and her
resources to meet those expectations. However, at the conclusion of
his work he attacks the picture of life satisfaction in as far as it is
linked with 'the myth of the golden years'. He argues that:

the image of life satisfaction is built on a single conception of
adjustment. To be adjusted in old age, it is implied, is to exhibit the
following behaviour: (1) above all, to be 'happy', (2) to be altruistic-
ally involved with younger persons, (3) to maintain a 'busy' everyday
life, and (4) to accept voluntarily the comparatively deprived social
conditions that exist for many aged persons.

In effect this conservative approach expects old people to adjust to
and be happy in situations that are demonstrably miserable and unsatisfactory. Dissatisfaction would be a more healthy response to such
conditions.

Provided it is not assumed that the life satisfaction index ought to
indicate high satisfaction, the test is a useful measure of an individual's perception of her situation. The particular test used in this study
was Life Satisfaction Index B (Neugarten et al., 1961; see pp. 120–1
below for example of use in this study).

This test is a shortened version of Life Satisfaction Index A. The
test has been criticised by Bigot (1974), amongst others, who considered
that a particular selection of these questions provided a fuller picture.
However Life Satisfaction Index B was used in this study because
it employs a number of open-ended questions, as well as being designed
so that it may be scored.

Both open-ended questions and scoring helped in understanding
Mrs Roberts's view of her life. Although she appeared to be managing

her life better than many residents since she was more active and lively, the Life Satisfaction Test showed her considerable dissatisfaction with her present life. In fact she scored 11 on the test and was below the average score for the home of 13.

Her responses to the first four questions clearly illustrate her feelings.

(1) *What are the best things about being the age you are now?*
It's a pity you have to get old. Why do you have to suffer? Go through a lot of aches and pains.
(2) *What do you think you will be doing five years from now?*
Kicking up the daisies.
(3) *What is the most important thing in your life right now?*
To get rid of my aches and pains.
(4) *How happy would you say you are right now compared with earlier periods of your life?*
Other periods were happier. Much of a muchness.

The test proved easy to use and the scoring range showed clear differences between residents. It was of value in testing out assumptions of contentment, as with Mrs Roberts, since some residents whom staff thought very happy scored low on the test. The other useful aspect was that the questions encouraged thoughtful reflection on the part of respondents.

### THE STUDY AND ITS DEVELOPMENT

The particular home to be studied was selected by the local authority. The main areas of consideration were that the home should be one with a stable regime, that the head should be agreeable to the scheme and that the home should be geographically convenient for me to reach.

The Pines is a purpose-built thirty-six-bedded establishment with twenty-four single rooms and six double. It is near the town centre and, as important, near a main access road to the town. There are shops and a pub in the immediate vicinity.

The building has stairs and a central lift. The six sitting areas, accommodating between four and nine residents, are open-plan. Downstairs there is also a kitchen, dining room, small staff room and an office. Upstairs there is a laundry and a sewing room. The bathrooms are mostly on the top floor; there are several lavatories on both.

On my introductory visit one of the senior staff explained that the home had been opened seven years previously as the first of three new homes to replace an old institution. All of the first thirty-six residents were transferred on one afternoon in two hours. Three of the present

Figure 3.1  *The Pines, ground floor*

Figure 3.2  *The Pines, first floor*

six female care assistants had worked in the old establishment, as had one male care assistant. The matron and one of the assistant officers were appointed to open the home; staffing increases had led to the appointment of two other assistant matrons, one full-time, one part-time. The historical context is important because it is easy to present a picture of an organisation as static, whereas those within the organisation may be aware of considerable changes over time.

At the opening of the home a senior staff member had been told by the welfare officer 'It will take ten years to get rid of the institution atmosphere' and, when I spoke to her, the staff member thought that was right. The staff who had transferred to the new home had been concerned for their jobs and for the changes that might be demanded of them. One of the significant changes for the senior staff had been the progressive reduction in working hours and the introduction of set 'times on'. 'It is more like a supermarket now' was the comment because of the regular change in staff. Senior staff were no longer necessarily around at times of illness or death. 'I never thought it would come to this' said a senior staff member.

### A synopsis of the study

The purpose behind this project was:

> To study a particular old people's home with the intention of making links between its practice and a typology of old people's homes worked out in advance, specifically to understand the attitudes to ageing of the people within the home, and interested parties outside, to see what relationships there are between attitudes to ageing and practice within a home.

The project covered eleven months and could be divided into three periods.

(1) *September–December.* At the start of this period in my research notes I used the word 'drift' to describe my involvement, with the idea of demonstrating being taken with the tide. At this time I needed to get to know people, to give clear messages about my purpose and to be around with different groups of people and at different times. In addition I began to look at the information available on various indicators (e.g. meal-times) so that I could relate The Pines to my typology. At the end of this time I met people who worked outside the home and developed an interview schedule for use with residents and a questionnaire to distribute to other groups.

(2) *January–March.* During this period I interviewed residents and produced and distributed the questionnaires which were given to staff, outside professionals and a few relatives.

(3) *April–July.* I started analysis of the questionnaires and produced reports for staff and outsiders and a summary report. Towards the end of this period I had the luxury of more free time in which I could take residents for walks or sit and chat. During the year I produced three newsletters for staff and residents.

*Methods used*

These were (*a*) participant observation, (*b*) interviews with residents (and a few staff), (*c*) a few written comments from staff and residents, (*d*) administration of life satisfaction tests to residents, (*e*) questionnaires to staff, relatives of residents, field social workers, other interested professionals (health visitors, doctors, nurses), (*f*) studying available records such as staff rota, menus, logbooks.

(*a*) *Participant observation.* The observer is not neutral and therefore measures need to be taken to focus and structure the observation. A first step is to specify one's own values. Some of my comments before starting were:

> My picture of old age includes life having some purpose; the potential for an old person to choose how he or she would live; the old being treated as responsible; some fear of increased dependence – especially physical disability (e.g. not being able to read), eneuresis, confusion. I find it hard to believe that sitting round and being bored is the result of real choice, nor do I believe in organised activities to anaesthetise and stop thinking. Neither forced inactivity nor forced activity can be right.
>
> Things that make me angry: staff being cruel, uncaring, laughing at or babying residents – and so creating the conditions they deplore; rigidity of routine; public living; boredom, loneliness, apathy of residents; lack of interest of staff; powerlessness of residents.
>
> Things I like: the possibility of privacy; concern expressed by gentleness; no bullying; the resident in control of the situation; enjoyment of life; death discussed and treated openly.

A second safeguard is to test findings against an established framework. (My framework was the table of models and the indicators.) While there are risks in participant observation it is often forgotten that there are risks in other methods. For example, even collecting statistics proceeds from a value assumption that such information is important.

Far outweighing the risks of participant observation, however, are the advantages – of understanding the meaning of a situation for the people involved, of discovering new perspectives, indeed, of finding that a new set of questions has to be examined.

Thus Miss Hutchins, a nearly blind resident, with severe walking difficulties, hobbled slowly back to the sitting room after lunch. A care assistant said 'Come on then, lift that right leg a bit' and the resident walked quietly by. She was regarded as a meek and contented person though often disoriented in space and time. In fact, having passed the care assistant she muttered: 'Does she think I do it on purpose? They'll find out when they are older.'

A second example illustrates the way a new area comes to be examined. I was sitting in the entrance hall before breakfast, while residents passed on their way to the tables. Mr Jepson came out of the lift and rested on his zimmer walking aid. He looked up at the slow-moving procession of people with sticks and zimmers. 'It's strange how it happens, you're all right one day.' This was the first pointer to the importance of considering adaptation to disability, as well as adaptation to residential living.

There is, of course, no way round the fact that the situation is altered by the presence of the observer. This must be acknowledged and the observer needs to use resources to minimise the effect, for example, by sitting outside a sitting area and recording movements, as well as sitting inside and joining in the conversation.

Another procedure is to record details of an incident and then get the differing explanations of people involved. Getting to know the observer over time will change the situation from one of guardedness to a situation where his presence, though noted, is not the most significant aspect in any interaction.

At the beginning I tried not to get too closely identified with any one group within the home. I joined senior staff for coffee-breaks, care assistants at lunch, went to each sitting area to meet residents. It is easy to forget the uncertainty of staff about what to do with me and the uncertainty of residents as to exactly what I was meant to be doing. A staff member recalled at the end of the study how fed up she had been when asked 'You'll take Mr Clough with you, won't you?' on my first afternoon. A resident at lunch was anxious that I needed help from the staff to find out what to do. Another explained my presence to a visitor by 'Oh, he's from college', which obviously explains everything! Similarly I was concerned about the impression I was making and the best way to record events.

I joined in as a staff member serving meals, taking round the drinks trolley, helping residents to stand and walk, making beds and, occasionally bathing. In this period I made sure that I was present early in the morning and in evenings and at night-time, as well as during the day.

It was more difficult to observe staff without my presence modifying behaviour. For example, I joined a care assistant bathing a resident and found the care assistant talking to me, when normally she would have conversed with the resident. Even following a member of staff round had its difficulties. I followed a care assistant round as she woke residents with a cup of tea. From one room the man said 'Come on, then'. 'No, not this morning' was the reply. And to me she said: 'They're funny some of them. He likes a kiss in the morning.' Presumably had I not been there, he would have had it.

Situations where I was not so conspicuously an observer provided more typical material. Serving in the dining hall it was easy to be working and also to be aware of the interaction of other people. An advantage of open planning for me was that I could be in one room and hear the conversation in another!

Another early problem was to communicate ideas to staff and residents since there were no staff meetings and no residents' meetings. The production of a news-sheet solved this and the first one of these aroused much more discussion than I had expected. Residents said: 'I read it and put it away to read again'; 'I like to see something that's independent'; 'I like reading things like that, very interesting'. There were comments too from staff – a cook said that it was very good but that I would never really know what the job was about until I had cleared up a mess after someone.

I used this and subsequent news-sheets to let people know what I was doing, and to propose ideas, such as residents writing about a day in their life.

Another difficulty with being an observer is to provide clear information about one's purpose. As I went round with one of the senior staff I had constantly to correct the picture that was being presented. 'Mr Clough is here to check, to find out ... ' Not surprisingly one person responded with 'You won't find anything to report on here'. I was aware from my introductory visit of the need for a precise form of words, which was 'to find out what it's like for people living and working in an old people's home'. Several months later, when I began interviewing residents, one resident was overheard to advise another not to take part on the grounds (imaginary!) that I was a Jehovah's Witness out to convert people.

Detailed notes were kept on incidents and conversation during each day. These were used both to record and to raise questions to follow up in other ways.

(b) *Interviews*.   The interviews with residents (see Appendix 2) were not tape-recorded. I had neither the resources to get all the interviews typed up nor the time to cope with the mass of paperwork involved. I made detailed notes, recording actual phrases where possible. This was helped by (1) the somewhat slower speech of many residents and (2) the fact that I paused to complete notes.

The full interview lasted between one hour and one-and-a-half hours. Nearly all of those residents interviewed were able to concentrate for this length of time, which surprised me. The interviews were spread over a period of several weeks. Only one person asked me when she was going to be seen and several, from comments fed back to staff, found it a difficult experience. One woman felt giddy after forty-five minutes, and never wanted to complete the interview; another stated that old people should not be harassed, that she should have been asked in advance (she had been but had forgotten), that she intended to consult her lawyer (a frequent riposte of hers). Needless to say that interview finished very quickly!

During the interview period there were thirty-nine people in residence (including one holiday visitor). Of thirty-nine possible interviewees, twenty-six were interviewed, three were judged too ill by staff, one was unable to speak, following a stroke and nine, for a variety of reasons, did not wish to be interviewed. This last figure, 23 per cent of the total available, is higher than I should have liked. I was aware of the residents' dependency and anxious to allow them a real choice. The only people I was prepared to persuade were two who said they had nothing 'good enough' to say. Of the nine who refused interviews, four had lived in the old workhouse. (There were nine residents from this workhouse – considering that one of these had also failed to complete the interview, 56 per cent of the ex-workhouse residents refused or did not complete interviews; three were very withdrawn, holding minimal conversations within the home; two felt they did not want to recall past problems.) Another person who refused was deaf and would not wear a deaf aid. I thought it would be too much for her, while the remaining three did not give precise reasons.

Interviews were held in residents' rooms except for one that finished in a pub since it was time for the interviewee's regular Guinness.

The interview schedule which I developed proved of more value in some parts than others. Multiple-choice questions were difficult to use. For example with question 21 about the aims of old age homes, I wanted interviewees to select one of four statements as the most important, or add others of their own. In fact hardness of hearing coupled with some difficulty in remembering all the items made it impossible to answer without considerable development of the question by me. This leads me to question the appropriateness of multiple-choice questions with old people and, indeed, the reliability of evidence drawn from such questions.

The questions that aroused the greatest response were those that asked for descriptions, in particular questions 11, 14 and 18: 'Do you remember how you came to think about admission to a home?', 'Can you tell me what happened when you first arrived?' (followed by prompts such as 'Did you come by car?'), and 'Can you tell me what you usually do during a day?' (with prompts such as 'Do you take long to get dressed?'). Questions that asked for direct answers sometimes had to be explained at great length and too many possible leads were then given about answering the question.

(c) *Written comments.* The few comments received from staff or residents contained some useful viewpoints. While this idea of diary writing is worth pursuing it is probable that it will only gain little response.

(d) *Life satisfaction tests.* These proved useful and have already been discussed (pp. 35–5 above).

(e) *Questionnaires.* Three different questionnaires were produced for staff (see Appendix 1), for interested outsiders and for relatives. Each had a different set of questions but had in common a series of statements about old age with which respondents were asked to agree or disagree.

Ten out of twelve staff completed questionnaires. Information was confidential, for staff were asked only to fill in their job descriptions, not their names. Matron and the assistant matrons used the term 'senior staff'.

I hoped to get information about: the perceived goals of the establishment; the satisfactions and dissatisfactions of the job; attitudes to old age and specifically to activity as a model of old age; those seen as the most popular, most unpopular and happiest residents; attitudes towards residential care; the importance attached to various tasks; possible changes in the running of the home.

Two sets of questions failed to get the desired response. In the first (questions 11 and 12) I asked which residents staff got on with best and which residents staff found least pleasant. These brought out a strong commitment to an often-stated policy within the home of 'no favourites'. While I knew this policy existed, I had not seen my question as being at variance with it. Three of four senior staff made specific comments: 'In my position I do not have favourites, they are all treated alike'; 'It is the policy of the home not to have favourites'; 'Definitely no favourites'. Those care attendants who made specific points stressed that 'I get on with everybody', 'Mostly get on with all of them', 'Everybody, including staff, can have an off day', 'Each has good and bad points'.

Only one person listed the people with whom she got on best, and she said that she could not say anyone was unpleasant. The question would have been better phrased in terms such as 'If you had a few minutes to spare to whom would you go and chat?', or 'Whom would you avoid if you could?'.

From the second set I hoped to get a picture of individuals' perceptions of the way they would age. However, the actual questions (25 and

26), 'Which resident do you think you will be like when older?'
and 'Which resident would you wish to be like when older?', probably
seemed too flippant.

The second set of questionnaires was sent to 'interested outsiders'.
Those approached were given a stamped addressed envelope, and this
was followed up by a further letter requesting return of the form. I
spoke on separate occasions to social services department staff, a GP
practice lunch-time meeting and the physician and ward staff from the
geriatric hospital.

Thirty-two questionnaires were returned: twelve from social services
department staff, seven from GPs and a physician, four from health
visitors, three from nurses at a geriatric hospital, three from 'friends'
of the home, two from district nurses and one from a county councillor.

Six relatives completed a third questionnaire. There was no easy
way of communicating with relatives. Several residents were concerned
not to worry their relatives with the questionnaire, even at times when
the relative had already indicated that she would complete the form.

(*f*) *Records.*   Immediate records of menus, drugs, or of residents'
ages and dates of admission were available. However, there was very
little written of any length. Official visitors recorded their visits and
made little comment, and the senior staff quarterly comments to the
social services committee were primarily about numbers, the weather
and outside events. The sparsity of information is itself a comment
on the style of running the home.

*The final stage.*   Research workers frequently collect a mass of
information from a wide range of people. The information is usually
confidential and gives to the research workers immense power. Re-
searchers must find appropriate ways of sharing that information and
should avoid producing a report after they have left an establishment,
when it may not be possible for them to discuss the findings.

I had agreed to feed back my ideas in the third phase of the study,
April to July. The production of the reports emphasised my committed
stance. While my task was to share the perceptions of the home, gained
from my own observations from interviews and questionnaires, the
selection of the material was bound to result from my bias. Therefore
my standpoint before going into the home (p. 39 above) needs to be
considered alongside any subsequent findings. Thus I was not neutral
simply by being a researcher.

Three reports were produced during the study period. The first, for
staff, was based primarily on staff responses to questionnaires but
included some details from interviews with residents and my own
observation; residents received a synopsis of this in the form of an
extended newsletter. The second report was for outsiders and brought

together perceptions of different people about admission and residential living. The third report, primarily for senior staff from the home and the department, highlighted some of the main findings while adding riders to earlier documents.

The first report had the most impact. I reported the feelings of staff and residents, described some events and offered explanations of events. My aim was to raise questions about practice but not to offer solutions. It was important to separate tasks since it was not for me but for others, the homes adviser and senior staff, to implement change if that was thought appropriate.

My objectives in producing the report were: (1) to produce a report that would get read – not too long, avoiding jargon, safeguarding confidentiality; (2) to build up a desire for change by shaking the complacency of staff; (3) to stress those areas which concern staff, for example, 'staff should not gossip'; (4) to take account of factors stressed by Rothman *et al.* (1976) which promote the preconditions for change; (5) to promote discussion amongst staff so that some norms might be exposed and questioned; (6) to stress specific areas of concern – (*a*) the admission process, particularly the loneliness, and the uncertainty at nights, (*b*) the powerlessness and dependence of residents, (*c*) the open discussion of residents and staff.

The production of the report and the reactions to it contain many of the central issues of the research. In fact it brought to a sudden halt the automatic acceptance of my presence within the home for I had been careful to avoid feeding back my impressions at an earlier stage.

For me it brought out the basic tensions between understanding what was happening and my lurking wish, which surfaced occasionally in various progress reports, to stop some things happening and produce change. The need for clarity of task pushed me towards the job of explanation of events but the frustration of not making statements about ways changes could take place was real, though I knew that if change was to occur it had to arise from and be implemented by those with responsibility for the establishment. In fact to be involved directly as a change agent it would be essential to be invited in for that purpose; change from the approach adopted in this study would be slower but might lead to a re-examination of methods in residential homes generally.

The report aroused mixed feelings among the staff. One care assistant was quoted as saying that she would never speak to me again. A senior staff member was described as 'unhappy or sad about it'. She was thought to be hurt because the residents had said the things they did. It was thought also that she saw nothing positive in the report. To me she said she felt that she might as well give up the work. Three members of staff regarded it as valuable, with material for discussion.

So I had to face the impact of my report but also the question, rightly raised by staff, as to the objectivity of the report. The incidents quoted were real and the statistics accurate, but they were selected to highlight certain aspects of residential living. Such selection is inevitable but it must take account of issues that concern other staff and residents as well as those noted by the researcher.

Two staff meetings held to discuss the report were chaired by the homes adviser. The reports – and meetings to discuss them – were the last of the formal aspects of the project.

*Personal summary*
The challenges of the first part of the study were about presenting myself and the details of method. So I was aware of the importance of confidentiality – and of saying repeatedly that I did not pass on information – of not becoming identified with one group, and of having a simple statement of purpose which also was repeated frequently. In terms of method I had to plan my time, work out a reliable form of note-taking and cover as many sources as possible – for example, circulars from county hall, minutes of Friends' meetings, lists of drugs, information on files – as well as discuss these items with staff. In fact it was a period of structure.

The structure continued into the period when developing the interview schedule and questionnaire. After that the structure was clear at particular moments – for instance, interviews, developing reports – but there was an increasing amount of informal involvement. In sitting with a group of residents or staff I was less concerned to steer the conversation to particular topics since I already had a mass of information on these.

One aspect that I was aware of from the beginning was that my presence might be intrusive. There is no doubt that residential institutions have been ready targets for research because of the captive situation of the resident. Therefore it is all the more necessary for the researcher to be sensitive to the feelings of residents.

A more complex problem arose when I started to produce progress notes on the research. To structure these notes I used the headings taken from the original analysis – control of life-style, with its various indicators, and attitude to ageing. The picture that emerged seemed a little distorted for, on reading the report, one person commented: 'I hope that I never have to go into a home then.' I felt that there were elements of the home that I had failed to capture. One possibility is that my involvement was already making it difficult for me to face up to the negative aspects of the home.

Another possibility needs careful consideration. This is that the variables selected are important, but on their own do not portray a full picture. Aspects such as security, dependability and continuity need far greater emphasis than they were given in this study. While they may be less easy to measure, such additional variables will demonstrate other aspects of life in a home. The gap was partly covered by looking for a range of opinion, from residents, staff and outsiders, and by examining the goals of the organisation but, nevertheless, failure to broaden the analysis will only perpetuate 'the myth of the evil institution'.

Another key area for me was the growing awareness that attitudes in old age are linked not only to personality characteristics but to other factors, in particular mobility and health.

An adult who has coped successfully with a variety of stress and change may still find it difficult to cope with whatever happens in old age. So the challenge is not only to theories that rate personality as the key variable to survival in old age; it is also to one's perception of one's own life when older. If I were so restricted in mobility that even getting to the lavatory became a wearisome effort, would I be as bitter as some of the residents. Certainly there were several who felt life was pointless or that they had been dealt a cruel hand by fate.

It should be stressed that the bitterness frequently had nothing to do with residential living – it had developed because life had become too much of a burden. I tried to reflect these feelings in a poem I wrote two months after starting the project. It expresses the futility or despair shown by a few residents and it illustrates also the effects on the observer. It is significant that the despair of the few may have a more marked effect on staff or visitors than the contentedness of others.

The poem starts from some typical comments of staff or residents.

'You've got your memories' – Yes, memories bring
Roses in December and children in old age.
But are we destined to become nothing but an album of past snaps?
'It's something to do' and 'it fills in time',
So, you knit and you knit and you knit,
Items that nobody wants.
There are feet that will not listen,
There are eyes that do not lead;
Bladders that are punctured and that leak.
Bodywork that's dented, hinges rusted up
Machines that can't be mended, only left to creak.
'Keep going', 'Keep trying', 'Keep moving' –
But 'For what?' I want to scream.

Two residents in particular, a man and a woman, faced a struggle, either with themselves or their legs, to keep walking, even with the aid of zimmer frames. It is in an area such as this that the perspectives of different groups are valuable. A geriatrician felt such a person must be kept mobile; staff differed in their response to the statement 'I can't walk today', depending on their own inclinations or that of senior staff. Some would wheel the resident in a chair to the dining hall; others would encourage the resident to walk one way and wheel him back in the chair; others would get the resident to walk both ways. Residents, watching a scene like this, would comment that it was for the resident's own good or think staff were being too strict. Underlying a lot of what was being said was a feeling, only occasionally made explicit, that a resident who lost all mobility would be transferred to a geriatric hospital.

Faced with the tears of the resident leaning heavily on the zimmer, the supposed struggle of the observer for objectivity is given up. (Perhaps it is put in abeyance since the preceding paragraph shows that in fact different perceptions of the situation were recorded.) While not opposing the wishes of staff, I would try to pre-empt such situations, or, if the individual was going to have to walk because staff said so, then ensure that I helped her as gently as possible. There remains no way of escape from the fact that the observer has no authority to change existing practices. It may be possible, when performing staff tasks oneself, to fulfil them in a different way. It would be pleasant also to be able to record that the result of the research was significant changes in practice, but it is too early to tell.

Some other points need mentioning. This was the first time I had seen the body of someone who had died; and I remember touching the body in the quiet of a small bedroom and talking with a staff member, for whom also this was her first sight of death.

From the interviews I became aware that residents needed help to get some things accomplished. There was a man who wanted to write but whose right hand was useless after a stroke; a woman who could not get adequate reception for her portable TV; several people frustrated by the life they were leading.

In the period after the production of the report I made it clear to staff that I was available to help in ways they wished and increasingly took an initiative in proposing things that I could do. So I took residents in wheelchairs round the town, to the pub and out in the garden; I took residents out with another member of staff for drives and a picnic; I helped the man already mentioned to learn to use a typewriter so that he could write letters; I took a discussion group of four residents when we talked about religion. All in all, I enjoyed the luxury of more time to sit and chat and do what I wanted.

The project came to an end with a special lunch. The home had won a 'Jubilee' turkey from *Woman's Own*, staff and residents sat down to eat it – at separate tables but for the first time staff were eating with the residents – the wine flowed freely and then I found myself feeling quite emotional during some speeches, and it all ended with hilarity as I was given the bumps.

A visitor quoted back at me a passage from my report to outsiders that spoke of the dominant picture of the home as 'a rather pleasant ordered calm'. 'Peace at last' said a senior staff member about my departure!

# Chapter 4

───────◆───────

# COMPARATIVE BACKGROUND
# INFORMATION

The thirty-six residents at The Pines comprise a small percentage of the total number of elderly people who live in residential homes, about 150,000. This group is itself only a small proportion, about 2 per cent, of the total number of people aged over 75 in the population. A brief discussion of such trends in the population and in residential institutions is included so that later information about The Pines may be placed in a broader context.

### OLD PEOPLE IN BRITAIN

The old (taken to be over 65, unless otherwise stated) are increasing both in number and as a proportion of the total society (see Figure 4.1). In this age-group the very old have increased at a faster rate than the younger and there are substantially more old women than men. In addition, women are more likely to be in need of services to help them since at all ages they are more dependent, less mobile and more likely to live alone. The very old are more likely to live in worse housing and to be poorer than other old people.

The growth in numbers of the old is apparent from the fact that

in 1901 there were 1½ million people aged 65 or more in a population of just over 37 million. In 1971 the respective figures were 7·1 million and 54 million. In percentage terms the over-65s had increased threefold from 4·0 per cent to 13·3 per cent, while the population was not quite half as much again in the same period. (Jeffrys, 1977)

Those aged 65 and over now constitute 14 per cent of the population of England and Wales. Two-thirds of this pensioner population are between 65 and 74 years and one-third are over 74 years. This latter group is composed of twice as many women as men and is where most of the real frailty is concentrated. Proportionately these older 'olds' are increasing at a faster rate. The women, mostly widows, are more dependent than the men who mostly have wives still alive. The male robustness reflects the fact that they are a group who have survived the critical middle-age years for men (35–55) when heart disease and cancer are major killers.

Figure 4.1 *Population aged 65 and over, England and Wales, 1951 and 1977*

In 1977 there were 824,000 men aged over 75, while there were over twice as many women: 1,780,900.

The trend for those aged over 75, and even more significantly for those aged over 85, to become an increasingly large proportion of all old people is expected to continue to 2001. Thus by 2001 women aged over 85 will be 11 per cent of all elderly women (cf. 1951: 4·8 per cent) and those aged over 75 will be 48 per cent of all elderly women (cf. 1951: 34 per cent).

The importance of these figures is demonstrated by comparing them with age- and sex-groups of those in need of services. It is women over 75, and in particular over 85, who make disproportionate demands for services.

Thirty per cent of elderly people live alone. Hunt (1978) shows that nearly 80 per cent of all those who live alone are women, and over 35 per cent are women aged 75 or more. Not surprisingly the chances of living alone increase with age, though women are more likely to live alone at any age. This is partly explained by the fact that men are more likely to be living with a younger spouse than women and that women live longer. Thus at 85 or over nearly 31 per cent of men are still living with their wives in a separate household. By contrast only 4·5 per cent of women over 85 are living with a spouse in a separate household. Sixty-six per cent of women aged 75 or over are widowed or divorced.

Hunt's study also shows that the 65–74 age-group are not much more disadvantaged physically than the age-group immediately beneath them. Indeed, people of 65–74 tend not to consider themselves old. However, the small percentage of this group who need services is still a significant total, for the group comprises about two-thirds of all elderly.

According to Hunt, 4.5 per cent of the elderly population were bed-fast or housebound and this increased to 20·6 per cent of the over-85 group. It is important to note that women at all ages were less mobile

Figure 4.2    *Age composition of local authority residential homes, England and Wales, 1966 and 1973. These figures include a small number who were supported by local authorities in voluntary or private homes*

than men. Power (1979) shows a significant drop in women's mobility between the 75–79 and 80–84 age-groups. For example, 61·7 per cent of women aged 75–79 could move freely, whereas only 41·9 per cent of the 80–84 group were able to do this.

Impaired mobility is a major cause of dependence on others. For those aged 75 and older, 7 per cent of men and 12 per cent of women cannot leave home unless assisted. A second major cause of dependence is confusion, although there is disagreement as to its meaning. Meacher (1972) argues that much confused behaviour arises from problems of social adjustment while others contend confusion is brought about by physical factors in the brain. Whatever the cause, the reality is that the confused elderly may need people in constant attendance to watch over them.

### RESIDENTIAL INSTITUTIONS

Of the 151,000 residents of old age homes in 1977, 30 per cent (46,000) lived in voluntary or private homes. Staff often state that their task has changed considerably – on admission residents are more handicapped, more confused than they used to be. It is said that residential homes are being asked to run as nursing homes or mini geriatric wards without the nursing resources of either of those establishments. How far is this an accurate reflection of the present state of residential homes?

### (1) *Age of residents*
Older residents are a growing proportion of those in old people's homes (see Figure 4.2). The major increase in numbers, even over a short seven-year period, has been for women over 75, in particular for women over 85.

### (2) *Dependence of residents*
It is much more difficult to chart increased frailty because measurements are far more reliant on the subjective interpretations of staff. This point is borne out in several places in the Census of Residential Accommodation. Some examples of the statements made about ways of collecting data are:

> The information provided by the homes relied upon the judgement and memory of those completing the forms and must therefore be treated with some caution. Respondents were asked to give details of the condition of the residents over the two weeks preceding the census and this meant that they should have accurate and up to date information about every resident. Opinions may have differed on definition of terms . . . (DHSS, 1975)

This point is emphasised again in relation to mental condition described as 'the least objective of the dependency measurements, as it is easily affected by observer bias; a particular resident is likely to be judged relative to the overall condition of residents in this particular home'. Finally, the development of measures of dependency is described as the most important area for improvement.

Nevertheless the survey does provide some information. Four factors were examined: continence, degree of mobility, self care and mental condition (see Table 4.1). Women, as would be expected, were less able to care for themselves than men. There were variations in levels of dependence between authorities (London boroughs had far higher proportions of dependent residents), but they do illustrate the large numbers of residents who are continent, able to walk around the home, and can feed themselves. Even with vague terminology like 'mental confusion' over half were judged mentally alert.

Table 4.1   *The abilities of female residents from local authority homes*

| Percentage of all female residents judged to be: | |
| --- | --- |
| Continent | 69 |
| Able to walk unaided | 44 |
| Able to feed self | 96 |
| Mentally alert | 52 |

*Source:* DHSS, 1975.

These figures, although dating back to 1970, are the most reliable available of the national scene. Hughes and Wilkin (1980) compare evidence from a range of sources. However, nearly all the material quoted is based on local survey and the DHSS (1975) survey is the only one which examines figures for England and Wales.

There is some possibility of comparison between Townsend (1962), whose fieldwork was carried out between 1957 and 1961, and the DHSS survey. Townsend found that 52 per cent of new residents needed little or no help to live in their own home; 61 per cent of women and 83 per cent of men were able to walk outside the building; 14 per cent were incontinent, 54 per cent needed help in bathing and 19 per cent in dressing. The DHSS (1975) survey shows an increase in incontinence and a dramatic fall in numbers able to bath themselves. The latter may be partly explained by the clear policy of most authorities that residents are to be supervised at bath-times which is likely to lead to undermining of residents' ability. Even allowing for this the change is significant, and particularly so in the light of the time that is given in staff hours to bathing residents. There are few residents in residential homes today who would need little or no help to live in their own homes.

A survey in East Sussex of applicants to residential homes examined capacity looking at nine areas concerned with personal care, physical health and mental health: 9 per cent had no incapacity and a further 16 per cent incapacity in only one area.

Table 4.2   *Category of residents in dependency areas, Cheshire*

|  | Mobility | Personal care | Mental state | Behavioural problems |
|---|---|---|---|---|
| Residents needing little or no attention | 82 | 63 | 68 | 70 |
| Residents needing attention | 18 | 37 | 32 | 30 |
| Total | 100 | 100 | 100 | 100 |

In Cheshire a survey examined the dependency of residents (see Table 4.2). Four areas were specified: mobility, personal care, mental state and behavioural problems. Residents were then divided into one of two categories: those needing little or no attention and those who needed attention (Kimbell and Townsend, 1974). This survey is useful because it followed up this material by examining how far residents had clusters of problems. Forty-three per cent of residents were shown to have problems in none of these areas – in other words they needed little or no attention to carry out functions in any of the four categories.

Brought together, these pieces of information suggest that residents are more dependent than was found by Townsend but that a substantial proportion of residents remains only minimally dependent. This is reinforced by the DHSS (1975) survey which found that nearly half of the residents required little personal assistance from the staff. The finding is extremely important in considering staffing and styles of living within the home.

(3)   *Marital status of residents*

However, it is useful to consider the other factors that may have contributed to admission since incapacity does not account for the total number of admissions. Age of residents has already been examined and it is clear that the very old are more likely to need residential care. Marital status is not mentioned by the DHSS or East Sussex surveys but the Cheshire survey shows the high proportion of widowed and single amongst the residents (Kimbell and Townsend, 1974). Ninety per cent of all residents were single or widowed, with 64 per cent of these being widowed (see Table 4.3).

Table 4.3   *Marital status of residents, Cheshire*

| | Single | Married | Widowed | Divorced | No reply | Total |
|---|---|---|---|---|---|---|
| Percentage of residents | 26 | 5 | 64 | 3 | 1 | 100 |

The proportion of single people is higher than for the population as a whole which is readily explained since without children they have a smaller network of relations on whom to call. Incidentally it should be noted that the number of children available to care for their parents has fallen with the fall in the birth rate. Evans (1977) shows that the number of potentially dutiful children available to support their parents fell by 19 per cent between 1951 and 1971.

(4)   *Previous residence*
There is considerable consistency between the DHSS (1975) survey and the Cheshire study. Of those in local authority homes, 30 per cent were admitted from hospital (DHSS, 1975). The full figures are given in Table 4.4.

Table 4.4   *Previous accommodation of residents in local authority homes*

| Previous accommodation | Percentage of residents in each category |
|---|---|
| Sheltered housing | 2 |
| Other housing – living alone | 24 |
| Other housing – living with others | 21 |
| Hotel/boarding house or lodging | 3 |
| Another residential home | 19 |
| Hospital | 30 |
| No settled residence | 1 |
| Total | 100 |

The large number – 19 per cent – who were admitted from other residential homes is largely accounted for by the closing of large, old institutions and the opening of new homes, though a smaller number would comprise those who were being transferred for other reasons – to move them nearer their former home or relatives, to cope with particular dependent residents in a more appropriate setting. The more surprising figure is that nearly one-third of all admissions came from hospitals. This indicates both the degree of handicap and the way in which a major break in the living situation appears to make the past pattern of caring an impossibility. Relatives may realise the effect on their own families of caring for a parent when the stress is removed.

Of course this does not make clear the previous residence of those who go into hospital. Townsend (1962) suggests that 50 per cent of all admissions were from people who were living alone – a much higher figure than for the elderly population as a whole. Harris comes to similar conclusions. She found that 47 per cent of all residents had been living alone and 41 per cent living with others. A further 69 per cent had lived in a hotel or boarding house and another 6 per cent with a spouse. The under-representation of the married is again demonstrated, together with the over-representation of those living alone.

## (5) *Reasons for admission*

Inevitably it is difficult to explain why people enter residential homes. A combination of factors so often exists that there is some distortion in listing the prime reasons. It has already been shown that incapacity on its own does not explain either application or admission to residential homes, although residents are more dependent than comparable age-groups in the general population (Harris, 1968).

Townsend's (1962) analysis has received substantial confirmation. Acknowledging that homes now take older and more dependent residents, there is widespread acceptance of additional factors that need consideration. Townsend listed the following:

Lack of close relatives and friends
Loss of supporting relatives
Separation from family and community
Consequences of isolation
Difficulties of living with the family
Homelessness
Housing conditions
Financial insecurity
Lack of domiciliary services

Perhaps the biggest change has been in the growth of domiciliary services. Many new residents have had considerable support from home helps and meals on wheels which contrasts with the picture painted by Townsend.

Harris has a much briefer section on reasons for admission. She states incapacity for self-care as the basic reason, often following illness at home or in hospital. Those who do not want to be a burden on children are another large group, and this may be associated with family friction. She cites 7 per cent of residents as wanting company – a positive reason for admission that stands out from the usual picture of lack of resources. Finally she mentions a small group with financial problems and a large group for whom housing is a major problem. This includes both poor facilities and homelessness.

The East Sussex survey found the two major reasons for admission were family problems and physical illness. It is interesting that those who stated physical illness were less incapacitated than any other group; it may be significant that 90 per cent of those who gave this reason were living alone and they may have felt an exaggerated sense of infirmity (East Sussex, 1975). The writers conclude that:

> there is evidence that factors such as homelessness, poor housing, isolation and loneliness and family stress were important and therefore that provision of services to combat these problems could have reduced admissions. These conclusions appear to follow fairly closely those of Townsend made over twenty years ago.

In a study of field social work Goldberg (1970) found only ten people who went into residential homes. Clearly this is too small for any firm conclusions but it may be significant that prior to admission six out of ten had said they were often or sometimes lonely and four were rated as discontented or openly unhappy by the assessor. This was a higher proportion than for those who remained in their own homes. Her concluding comment is: 'Thus in this tiny group it looks as though social reasons, both situational (housing) and personal, rather than incapacity in itself, are associated with entering a home.'

## (6)  *Planning and choice*

Admissions result, then, from a combination of stress factors. There is a hint from Harris that a small percentage of people wanted to go into a home for the company they would find but most writers pinpoint problem areas. This method of analysis seems appropriate for it matches the way most residents respond to questions about admission and illustrates the normal pathway to a residential home. A conglomeration of problems results in a crisis; the crisis leads to re-evaluation of the situation with the consequence of admission to a home. While for many admission may be *the best choice of living arrangement that is available*, it is almost never part of a planned change of life in old age.

There are exceptions to this. Some people do plan for a stage of life when they will need more support and then they have a choice available. They may get a friend, relative, or companion to live in; they may move to a smaller, more convenient house; some people plan to move to a private hotel; others buy flats in housing associations where support is available and a few plan to move to a voluntary or private home for the old. There is virtually no planning for entry to a local authority home because the resources are too scarce and are used to meet whatever is assessed as the greatest need. The possibility of admission at an earlier age to a voluntary or private home makes planning more realistic.

### (7)  Building programmes

Poor housing conditions are often a factor in necessitating residential care. The standard of housing provided by residential homes has shown a dramatic improvement. Indeed, one of the most consistent and expensive trends in social services must be the building of new homes for the old since 1948, but in particular since 1958. The major change has been in building over a thousand new medium-sized homes in England and Wales. In 1959 there were 443 medium-sized homes; *by 1973 there were 1,806*, a growth of over fourfold. In 1959 42 per cent of residents were living in large homes (over seventy places) with only 31 per cent living in medium-sized homes (thirty-five to seventy places). By 1973 77 per cent of residents were living in medium-sized homes and only 12 per cent in large homes. The change is all the more amazing when it is remembered that total numbers of residents grew from 60,900 to 100,400.

These medium-sized homes accommodated far more residents in single bedrooms – in 1970 30 per cent of all residents in local authority homes had single bedrooms with a further 32 per cent in double rooms. A DHSS Building Note in 1973 suggested that a maximum of one bedroom in nine should be a double room and all the rest be single rooms. This has not been achieved, but significant progress has been made. A further point in the Note is that there should be one WC for every four beds, and in 1970 only 30 per cent of homes met these requirements.

There is a basic tension between raising standards in existing homes and building new homes, and this is emphasised by the large sums of money that have to be spent to keep abreast of changes in fire regulations.

### Staffing

Between 1966 and 1973 the number of residents increased by 39 per cent. In the same period the number of senior staff (matrons, wardens and their deputies) increased by 54 per cent and the number of care assistants by 69 per cent. These increases are in whole-time equivalents, not gross numbers, so they are real increases. This means that there has been an increase in real terms in the numbers of staff (full-time or equivalents) that has exceeded the increase in the numbers of residents. However, it must be noted that the average number of hours worked per week has decreased in the same period so there has been little improvement in the number of hours of staff time available per resident. The ratio of senior and care staff to residents was 1:4·7 in local authority homes for the elderly. Interestingly voluntary homes had a slightly worse ratio of 1 : 5·3, but this was compensated for by more domestic staff, and they had less dependent residents.

There has been little increase in the numbers of qualified staff between 1960 and 1970. In 1970 83 per cent of local authority senior and care staff held no qualifications. Nearly 90 per cent of those qualified held a nursing qualification. Over half of those with non-nursing qualifications had attended only a fourteen-week course. So there were very few with any social work qualification.

Figure 4.3  *Population of The Pines, Somerset, and all local authority residential homes, 1966, 1973 and 1977*

## THE PINES AND SOMERSET OLD AGE HOMES

The proportion of older residents in Somerset old age homes has increased in line with the national average (see Figure 4.3).

Table 4.5 shows the previous residence of those admitted to Somerset residential homes in 1976–7. It is apparent that more people in this sample were admitted from hospital than in the DHSS survey in 1970 (38·5 per cent compared with 30 per cent).

Table 4.5    *Previous accommodation of those admitted to Somerset homes, 1976–7*

| Previous accommodation | Percentage of residents in each category |
|---|---|
| Sheltered housing | 7·0 |
| Other housing – living alone | 17·7 |
| Other housing – not living alone | 7·0 |
| Friends, relatives | 19·3 |
| Hospital: general | 14·7 |
| geriatric | 18·3 |
| psychiatric | 5·5 |
| Local authority home | 6·1 |
| Other home | 2·8 |
| Other address | 1·5 |

Dependency trends in Somerset can be compared for 1970 and 1978 (Somerset County Council, 1978). The numbers of residents who were substantially dependent remained the same, at 15 per cent of all residents. However, there was an increase in those moderately dependent from 40 to 50 per cent of all residents. Significantly most of this shift in overall dependency levels is attributable to residents aged 85 years or over. It is this age-group which has experienced the greatest shift from 'minimally' to 'moderately' dependent.

The differing dates of available figures have not allowed a direct comparison between the Somerset and the national figures on dependency. However, it is useful to see the figures for Somerset alone (Table 4.6).

Table 4.6    *Somerset long-stay residents' self-care abilities, 1978*

| | Dressing | Washing hands and face | Bathing | Use of WC or commode | Combing/ brushing hair | Feeding self |
|---|---|---|---|---|---|---|
| Alone – no difficulty (percentage) | 54 | 62 | 10 | 69 | 70 | 84 |

My period of study at The Pines was a year before this survey. Similar patterns were apparent at The Pines, though in a small home the figures in any box might change markedly from week to week.

Thus in so far as comparison is possible between all local authority homes and those in Somerset, the trends appear remarkably similar.

# Chapter 5

———◆———

## GOING INTO A HOME

### INTRODUCTION

There are, then, an increasing proportion of women over 85 who are residents in homes but such trends do not explain why some 85-year-old women apply for and are admitted to residential homes and others do not. The most comprehensive study examining this is one by Tobin and Lieberman (1976) in America. After a thorough review of other findings and a well-constructed research programme that was detailed in method and looked for changes over time, they emerged with the following conclusions. 'There is little reason to doubt that a wide array of types of people apply to and become residents of homes for the aged . . .'

They consider three variables to be important in explaining the reasons for entering a home: 'personal deteriorative changes in the older person, the inability or unwillingness of responsible others to offer the care that they or the respondent perceive to be required and the inability of the current system of services to assure independent living'.

Of particular importance is their finding 'that factors other than personality types must be used to explain why some older people and not others apply for admission to residential homes'. This is vividly illustrated by their case studies which show *over time* how individuals responded to changed circumstances. Events, such as death of a significant person or physical deterioration, might change people's attitude to life.

It has already been stated that an individual rarely plans in advance to enter a local authority residential home. The result of changed circumstances — of particular clusterings of events — is admission to a residential home. In this process the old person rarely initiates discussions with the social services department, the body responsible for running the home. Townsend (1962) writes: 'It was somewhat surprising to find that comparatively few of the new residents in our sample had acted on their own behalf and many of the local welfare agencies which might have been expected to play an important role in fact played a small one.' He found that it was the doctor, whether in hospital or general practice, who frequently played a significant first step. He continues: 'The old people did not take the same view as others of the conditions in which they were living and of the attractions of residential care. Doctors, for example, often told them that it was not in their best interests to remain in insanitary houses, and relatives argued that they should not live alone any longer without adequate help.'

### THE INFLUENCES OF THE DOCTOR AND SOCIAL WORKER ON ADMISSIONS

The doctor had been a significant person in seventeen of twenty-six admissions in the present study. This figure would certainly be higher if information were more precise: for example, some of the ex-institution residents did not remember who had been involved in arrangements, while one confused woman did not think she was in a home at all. In eleven of twenty-six admissions the doctor is reported as having *instigated* the process.

> The doctor asked me a year before I came in. 'Not yet', I said.

> The doctor said I had to give up. I had mixed feelings.

> The doctor said, 'You can't carry on like that'. It was a bit of a shock.

> The doctor suggested it. My daughter would have had a breakdown.

The doctor is the professional who comes into contact with the largest number of old people. There may well be others, home helps, district nurses, social workers, who have more intensive contact with *certain* of the elderly, but the doctor has the wider range of contacts. He also has more status than the other group and people *as patients* have become used to accepting recommendations. The doctor has also become used to *making* recommendations. Nevertheless the frequency with which the doctors had suggested admission to residents, and the authority given to their pronouncements, surprised me.

When social workers were already in contact with the person, as was the case with two women who were registered blind, the social worker was as likely to be chosen for help as the doctor. Relatives mentioned consultation with a social worker as much as with a doctor, presumably because social workers are more involved with detailed planning of admission. When consulted, social workers were less likely than a doctor to suggest admission to a residential home.

It is sometimes assumed that doctors are unwilling to supervise old people who are at risk in their own homes and that they too readily suggest the old go into a residential home. Social workers, on the other hand, give over-riding consideration to independence when perhaps the struggle of daily living *restricts* independence. Doctors, who see more of the struggles of the very frail old, in this study took a more negative attitude to old age than other groups (see p. 170 below), seeing it as more dreary, less of an opportunity to do new things, more boring and more depressing. There may be more times when doctors appropriately question whether the old should stay in their own homes than social workers may acknowledge.

> The doctor advised me to go into a home. I talked to my family who didn't want to hear of it. They didn't want to see my side. I had a home help three mornings from eight-thirty to ten a.m. but then had to manage on my own. I did the cleaning and the fires; lugging coal was a problem. I could manage the meals, and did the washing up. Some days I felt I didn't know how to carry on. My family didn't want to part with me. Brother would come and see me most mornings, would bring in a bucket of coal. There was no bathroom; the toilet was downstairs.

In this situation Mrs Richardson was living on her own, housing was restrictive, she received considerable support from home helps and had regular contact with her family. Nevertheless, *'some days I felt I didn't know how to carry on'*. There is no easy solution to her problem. Since she lived in the country rehousing would involve a move away from her family and it is impractical to consider a greater range of domiciliary services. For her the best alternative was a residential home. Any choice had severe limitations and this will need to be remembered in later sections when the restrictions of residential living are examined. These must be balanced against the restrictions of other styles of living.

It would be useful to have more detailed information than was available from this study about the actual knowledge of all parties (doctors, social workers, relatives, prospective residents) about particular homes. How far are major life-decisions for the elderly made on casual recommendations from others?

While the great demand for local authority homes makes choice *between* homes difficult, the choice between staying in one's own home and moving to a residential home should be made with detailed knowledge. For those who plan to pay for residential accommodation there is more choice, but I suspect many decisions are still made on casual hearsay. Two themes are worth pursuing further: the *routes* by which different groups of the elderly approach residential homes and the ways in which people may find out about styles of living in old people's homes.

The perceptions of different people about strengths and weaknesses of residential living (see pp. 173–6 below) are also important influences on the decisions of the old. The evidence in Chapter 11, though from only a very small sample, suggests that doctors were less aware of the psychological aspects of entering a residential home than were social workers.

### REASONS FOR ADMISSION

It was shown earlier that ten interviewees had lived with others before admission. These living arrangements broke down for a variety of reasons, of which the most significant was hospitalisation either of the old person or some crucial person in the care-system. In two cases the caring daughter went into hospital, in another two the old person. The spell in hospital would seem to have made a tenuous situation impossible. Harris (1968) makes a similar point.

> Quite often this stage [of not being able to look after oneself] is reached immediately after a spell of illness, treated either at home or in hospital. Doctors in hospital often recommend a residential place before discharge where an elderly person lives on his or her own, particularly when housing conditions are bad. A number of the elderly go into residential accommodation because their doctors recommend it as they might fall when on their own, or because they are advised against being on their own at nights.

However, these points would seem to apply more to an individual living alone. The significant fact in relation to the care-system is that the problems related to the illness are coupled with an opportunity to demand a change. Hospitalisation is conspicuous and can become the event that leads to change.

Of the remainder who lived with others: one person's daughter was said to be on the verge of a breakdown; the 73-year-old resident housekeeper of another needed a rest; in another case the caring daughter was moving away; while one woman felt she was in the way of the grandchildren; and one woman who was living with a friend of a similar age found she could no longer do enough herself to make the situation viable.

Those living alone gave the following as reasons for admission: six spoke of problems of managing the house 'It was getting beyond me, I couldn't get upstairs'; 'I kept on till I couldn't cope – I was spoiling cooking pans'; two mentioned poor housing, in particular dampness; one could not manage following an accident; two were thought too confused to continue managing (social work report); one was considered 'at risk' with respect to health (social work report).

Several residents stressed that they preferred a residential home to living with children because they did not want to be a burden, nor did they wish to feel restricted.

I wasn't getting any better; I was relying on my family so much and they had to lead their own lives.

I've only got a daughter. I didn't want to be any burden.

I made up my mind too quickly. I had my daughter to think about.

One woman described why she stopped living with a relative:

I lived with my husband's grand-daughter for nine years. She was very kind, had two children. I used to get in their way; it wasn't pleasant for the children or the parents. 'Don't get in Nan's way' she used to say.

I lived with my youngest son for twelve months. 'I don't want to interfere in your life; I'd rather go in a home' I said.

I had thought I might live with my son. They had only three bedrooms and one large sitting room downstairs. The children needed the beds. My daughter-in-law likes meeting people and going out – she goes out to work all day. My youngest son's marriage had broken up, my daughter only had a flat. I didn't want to go to the children if I was able to go somewhere else; I don't want to be a burden.

I couldn't go to my son. They are both out at work. Young couples have things all special. I wouldn't go there in any case – my daughter-in-law is very particular – she has got everything all new. I'd feel all on pins about knocking things over, marking the carpet.

There are two different strands in the reasons given for not being with a family. One strand acknowledges that the old person may be in the way of the family and risk being a nuisance, while the second stresses the wish not to be a burden and leads to an emphasis that the decision was that of the resident not of the family. Thus Mrs Smith emphasised that her family wished her to stay in her own home, as did Mrs Williams and Mrs Richardson. The fact that these three were all living alone prior to admission may be significant.

Tobin and Lieberman (1976) contend that the 'resident-to-be cannot afford to be rejected because the home has been determined to be the best, if not the only, solution available. To handle the rage and to maintain self-esteem, the resident-to-be usually emphasizes that the decision to apply to the institution was wholly his own.' They suggest that for some people this may be a reasonable mechanism for coping with anger and fear.

However, their proposition does presume that most old people have this fear of rejection. Twenty-six per cent of a group they interviewed on the waiting list for admission to homes introduced the issue of rejection when discussing changes in relationships. The difficulty is that, unless the fear of rejection can be demonstrated from other sources, there is a danger of assuming that all those who state that they themselves decided to enter a home are employing defence mechanisms.

An important dimension that was mentioned earlier is the part played by the professional workers in influencing decisions. Therefore it is essential to know any differences between groups of workers about reasons for admission and the purpose of residential homes.

In this study those working with the elderly in the town were sent questionnaires. The opinions about reasons for admission are shown by answers to two questions which distinguished between the main reasons that necessitated admission and factors that changed a viable situation into one that necessitated admission.

Two major sets of reasons for admission were given: (1) the inability of the old person to cope and (2) an inadequate support-system. Twenty-one people mentioned the inability of the individual to manage. This included 'frailty', 'self-neglect', 'danger to self', though many used the phrase 'unable to cope' which presumably meant an inability to complete the daily tasks of living. Most groups of professionals mentioned this as a reason.

An inadequate support-system was noted by nineteen people. Here comments included relatives or neighbours being unable to cope, friction or breakdown between some members of the household, death of a spouse – all of these suggested a breakdown in an existing support-system. The absence of any support-system was a reason given by six people. Significantly health visitors and social workers concerned with social situations all gave considerable weight to an inadequate support-system, whereas doctors did not. The nearest comment by a doctor was 'no care or supervision at home'.

Poor health was a third area mentioned. This included immobility, mental and physical disability, malnutrition, illness and recovery from illness, and was mentioned by eleven people from all professional groups.

Isolation was mentioned in five replies. This covered lack of contact with others, lack of interest in life and loneliness. Other reasons given included accommodation, the preference of the individual and no other alternative.

The inadequacy of the support-system was given even greater weight when considering reasons that made a situation intolerable. Twenty-eight responses mentioned insufficient support or support that had broken down through death, moving away, or changing expectations of the 'care-takers'. The circumstances detailed about the individual old person are similar to responses to an earlier question, though deteriorating health and illness or accident were given very much greater emphasis. Surprisingly doctors rarely mentioned health problems as the factor that changed a viable situation into one that was not; it was health visitors, followed by social workers, who saw these as most significant.

In fact there seem two basic patterns. In one situation the elderly person goes to live with a son or daughter and the stress of the physical caring or emotional involvement become too great, a fact which is often brought home when the situation is temporarily changed through hospital admission.

In the second set of circumstances, an inability, or an unwarranted struggle, to complete basic household tasks leads to application to a residential establishment. The professional groups have a similar picture of the first pattern to those involved, but attach much less weight to the decreasing mobility of the elderly than do the elderly themselves.

### OPINIONS AS TO SUITABLE AND UNSUITABLE RESIDENTS

It is important also to find out the characteristics of those who are seen as suitable or unsuitable candidates for residential homes, since it has already been shown how influential is the professional in steering people towards residential homes. Respondents claimed that they would *discourage*:

(1) Those able to care for themselves (ten responses). People who were coping adequately or were fit enough to stay active were mentioned under this heading.

(2) Those seen as independent (eight responses). 'Independence' was cited frequently, for example, 'those who were not lonely and valued independence'. A stronger statement was 'those with sufficient backbone to go it alone'.

(3) Those with unsuitable characteristics (seven responses). This included both people 'who would not mix well' and those regarded as difficult, awkward, or anti-social.

(4) Those with adequate support (seven responses). This group comprised those cared for by family, or other helpers such as neighbours or home helps.

(5) Those seen as too sick (four responses). This was used to indicate those too sick to be in a residential home, but it was difficult to define the boundary.

Other responses included 'those who could afford private homes who would not fit into a local authority home', 'those expecting a five star hotel'.

The picture of those seen as suitable for a residential home is far less clear. It indicates the lonely, those at severe risk, those with deteriorating health, those unable to care for themselves, the dependent and those without support. A large number (nineteen responses) mentioned one of these last three categories but the responses do indicate wide differences of understanding about the need to enter a home. For example, some thought a residential home was needed for those unable to care for themselves (a reply which would fit the perception of the old about reasons for admission); others coupled this with lack of support, while a further group added the word 'dependent'. While the responses do not make clear whether dependence is viewed in physical or emotional terms, the high rating given in the earlier question to those with 'backbone' staying out suggests that dependence is viewed in personality terms and negatively. The single word used most commonly in this answer was *lonely* – a clear statement that respondents would encourage the lonely to enter a residential home.

In effect the combination of factors that lead to admission has been illustrated. Residents are likely to be unable to look after themselves *and* to be lonely, or psychologically dependent, or without support. The different perceptions about the suitability of applicants are crucial because most residents had not considered admission before it was suggested to them. Since places in residential homes are a scarce resource some sort of rationing is inevitable. One aspect of that rationing is the influence of the professional worker but the discussion above has shown how haphazard that influence is. In considering which people should be encouraged to enter residential homes there was a very wide spread of answers though some clustering of views around the lonely and the immobile was apparent. This emphasises the dilemma between providing residential homes for those who will enjoy and benefit from them or those who could be said to 'need' residential accommodation, because they are at risk. If the first option is taken the anti-social or awkward are excluded, if the second these same people are included because they are 'in need of' a place in a residential home. While some respondents would consider the awkward or anti-social for residential homes, most would not. Different professions gave different answers.

### ALLOCATION

Doctors stressed that they would discourage the fit, the independent, the self-sufficient, and would encourage those who were frail, forgetful, had decreasing mobility and those with poor support-systems. Probably because they were farther removed from management responsibilities they gave less attention than social workers to excluding those with unsuitable characteristics, nor did they consider placing those who would benefit from residential living.

Two aspects must be separated out. The first is the process which leads to application, the second is the way in which decisions are made about allocating places. In the first stage doctors have been shown to have significant influence, and the opinions of professionals as to who ought to go into a home are important. While doctors may influence significantly which people apply for residential care, it is the social services department that allocates vacancies. The local area team of social workers discussed at a meeting held with the writer the way allocations were made. A health and mobility scale had been used in the past to assess priorities for admission. Recently so many applicants had maximum points on the scale that it no longer discriminated effectively. For permanent admission they excluded those who were frequently incontinent, those unable to move around even with a walking aid and the mentally confused where this was likely to lead to a serious management problem. They gave priority to a person living on her own.

The pressures placed on the area team were considerable and show the marked contrast with most other residential provision under social services' control. While there is a shortage of places for any sort of residential home the demand for allocation comes from other professionals – for example, in the case of an unruly child from the school, from other social workers. With the elderly, the social services' department is subject to considerable pressure from relatives, doctors and even the elderly themselves. The local newspaper is scanned and the announcement of a death at an old people's home is followed by phone calls requesting that a particular individual be allocated the place. In addition individual social workers will be pressing the cases of particular clients.

The social workers in this team stressed the right of individuals to decide their own style of living even if it did not seem satisfactory to the social worker. They would uphold this principle in the face of their own doubts and pressure from neighbours or relatives. However, they would not face the threat of medical resources being pulled out, although they would endeavour to get a second opinion from the community physician.

This shows some of the factors considered by one area team of social workers. Other studies (East Sussex County Council, 1975) have shown that different divisions within one authority may have different methods of assessing whether an elderly client requires residential care. 'The amount and depth of information required to be provided by social workers varied considerably and so did the informal unwritten criteria applied.'

There have been attempts to standardise procedures within an authority. One such (Davies and Duncan, 1975) drew up minimal criteria for admission and a system of weighting applications. The establishment of minimal criteria (which include the wish of the elderly person to go into a residential home) demands that domiciliary services have been considered and that assessment is structured around certain headings. The priority groupings list six sets of social circumstances (housing, tension in household, at risk, disabled, mental disturbance, hospital) and gives four gradings of priority in each situation.

To return to the particular situation of this study, the process of application involved the applicant being interviewed by a social worker, and seeing a booklet produced by the local authority which attempts to answer some of the questions people may have about residential homes. Social workers felt the booklet was more help to relatives than to the elderly themselves.

## MOVING IN – RUSHED DECISIONS AND LOSS OF POSSESSIONS

Except with urgent admissions the prospective resident has the opportunity of getting to know the home through a short stay or day care. Of twenty-six interviewees, five had been transferred from the old institution. Of the remaining twenty-one, seven remembered holiday visits, two had paid short afternoon visits, four stated that they did not want a trial because they knew the home, eight offered no information about this.

There was no correlation between residents who were most satisfied with current life-style (as shown by the life satisfaction index) and prior visiting to the home. What did emerge is that several people knew of the home from visiting friends, from coffee mornings, from singing in a visiting choir. So it is useful to consider ways in which the local community may get to know a home. Though a short visit is better than none at all, its unsatisfactory nature is shown by one resident who thought after the visit that she was to have a little flat on her own.

The extent to which a resident felt that she had influenced the decision to come into a home was closely related to life satisfaction scores. Those who stated they had decided to come in, often ignoring the wishes of their families that they stayed out, were more likely to be satisfied than those who came from care-systems that had broken down. This fits with Tobin and Lieberman's findings discussed earlier, though it does not assume such choice to be the result of a defence mechanism. In particular those who felt the decision had been made *for* them were likely to have low satisfaction scores. A man was unable to remember anything about coming in: 'See my daughter' he said – and he still hoped, totally unrealistically, to return home.

'I wanted to be independent, I don't know why I came in, I don't know why she [her daughter] got me in' said a woman, and this situation illustrated the pressure that may be applied, particularly to rush a decision. 'My daughter spoke to the social worker about it. "I've got the social worker coming in, what do you think about going into a home?" she said. It was a shock to me, I only had about a fortnight to decide.'

For others the pressure related to having to settle affairs too quickly, even after making the decision to go on to a waiting list for admission. Inevitably vacancies could not be planned but a typical response was 'when it came, it was sudden'. Interviewees described asking for more time and a staff member commented that most people take a long time to plan moving home to a new area whereas the elderly are expected to settle everything in a few days.

An extreme example is that of a woman on a fortnight's holiday visit to see if she liked the home. At the end of a week a death occurred in the home and it was decided to offer the vacancy to the holiday resident.

Her account of the incident is interesting.

Last May [eight months before] I had a fall. The doctor said 'Wouldn't you like to go into a home?' I didn't think anything more about it until just before Christmas [only one month before the interview]. Then a gentleman came to see me, he might have been from the housing, he took notes. He said that there was a bungalow or flat going empty. 'No, if I give up my home, I'll go to The Pines', I said.

Then a social worker came, the week before Christmas, and brought a card to say the dates [for holiday visits]. Then she came last night to say there was a room vacant, but I'd have to share. I got Matron to show me the room – it was rather small, I'd want to bring my own commode. What room is there to put things in? The social worker said I couldn't bring in much, so I'll leave it till I go and see. She said if I didn't take this opportunity there would be a wait. I wanted to come in before the winter but this is rather sudden.

She decided to take the offer of a place and was asked to take up residence the following Monday, six days after the first discussion. She was able to get this put back a week. There had only been about five weeks from the first serious discussion of admission to a home with a social worker. Clearly the administrative need to maintain high occupancy rates may be at variance with the needs of the elderly to have time to adjust to changed situations and time to make decisions.

The uncertainty of this resident about what she could bring in was common and several people wished they had brought in more. Other comments were:

I didn't know what to bring in. She told me, the welfare person, I could take a table or rug, could take an ottoman. I sold lots of things privately.

My daughter said 'Oh you don't want to have a lot of stuff'.

I took what I wanted. Brought my work box. The chest and carpet I bought since. Didn't want to bring in anything else, wanted to forget. I didn't want to be cluttered up, I get around better. I put my photos away. (A blind woman)

The dominant picture prospective residents appear to have had was that it was reasonable to bring in a commode and one or two small items. Some had not even understood this. There are six double rooms in the home and a new resident always shares a double room. This means that there is not much space for anything other than a commode and small items. Added to this it is made clear to residents that domestic staff like a tidy room without too much clutter around.

Others discovered that, when they moved into a single room, things for which they then had room had been given away.

'I gave away a lot of things that I wish I hadn't – lots of little things. I didn't know you could put in your own furniture.'

The rooms of two residents were a contrast. One decided to bring in a lot of things and got rid of those she didn't want; another was where a woman was unable to sell her house and therefore was able to go back to collect other things she wanted. Her room was a great contrast to every other one. It was cluttered up with bits of furniture, ornaments and a large sewing machine. A senior staff member said: 'She moves the furniture around and has it in her own individual style. The girls [domestics and care assistants] don't like it but I think if she can't get in it to sleep, that's her problem.'

Finally, two observations suggest that given active encouragement some more reticent residents might hang things up. In both cases the rooms were spartan with nothing around. One man showed me treasures of his in the wardrobe – photos of his parents' marriage – and described some fretwork and a mirror that had been stored upstairs and he'd never had up. This was similar to an experience when the room of a man who was leaving for hospital was being cleared up. He had nothing of his own around. Now from drawers and the wardrobe there turned up old photos of the man, young and handsome in the army, and an intricate woven sampler presented by his firm and wishing him well on retirement. Several staff members commented how easy it was to see only the present person, a shell of a man constantly wet and dirty, and to forget that he had been someone with a real past.

It is comparatively easy to remedy this by giving time to hanging up pictures. However the problem with furniture is far more complicated. Ideally residents need time to adjust to their new life-style before disposing of possessions. Modern purpose-built homes have little space for storage, and families, if not the resident, are anxious to tidy up the house the resident is leaving. Some social workers (at a meeting with the author) wondered whether it might be possible to find anywhere else to store furniture.

## FIRST IMPRESSIONS

The following extracts give a picture of the memories of residents about the first few days.

Three people remembered coming from the old institution.

I didn't like the thought of going to the institution. I had heard so much about it, we used to call it the union. Had to go because there was nowhere else to go. The food was nice when we came here, had more meat.

I liked it coming here. A man came and showed me up to my room, a nice young fellow. The WVS brought our luggage, it was like a railway station. A good job we came here, nobody to interfere with us. It's nicer, happier, more at home.

I didn't want to come here. The other place was more comfortable, warmer and no draughts. You need doors here. There were no men there. The cooking is marvellous here, atrocious there.

This is a palace compared to that. People were happy there, heartbroken to leave [though she went on to say how much better the move was].

Others had come from their own home or hospital.

I had a good idea of what to expect, nothing was different from what I knew.

The welfare brought me. I came just in time for lunch. I have been in a good many places, I soon fell in.

I was excited about coming in. Surprised to see such a wonderful place. People were treated better than I expected. A social worker brought me in with my luggage. Matron met me and took me up to my room, an attendant unpacked and put everything away.

They greeted me and I felt pleased with the way I was greeted. Took me upstairs with my case. I didn't mind sharing a room because I felt there was someone to guide me with the lift. Brought me back down and I had a meal at dinner time . . . others kept me in conversation; I felt it wasn't too bad. The Pines felt like a home. The difference from your own home is not working any more.

The most important thing was feeling comfortable – nothing to worry about; able to rest; done my duty; surprised at such a place.

Another talked about the people – their moans and groans.

It's a different atmosphere. Mrs X is boss of the show. I had been in for a visit but when I came in it was sudden. I think a lot about what I left behind – little treasures, saving old-fashioned things, magazines, a favourite chair, a knife and cup, not a plastic mug; I use my own mug a lot. I miss the life around my home – everyone was jolly.

It's living with other people, not your home. You have to have what food is given; to make life decent you have to swallow so much.

It was not as hard for me as for some people, I was used to institutions. Had to be sure stuff was marked. The cooking is all right but it's not like home. I miss the salt, though sometimes I don't.

I miss the phone, my own possessions, miss the friends from home, the control of the TV.

I miss my independence. I didn't like it for three months till I got into the rhythm. Very handy, rather like it now – terrific things to get used to. I was used to deciding things for myself – cleaning, sewing when I wanted. I'd been in the army, used to discipline – the feeding arrangements didn't upset me. Living with other people is difficult, I can't describe it.

I came in June. It was a Monday morning, raining. It's nice with friends all round now. I used to clean my bedroom, make bed, cook the dinner. I miss not having enough to do, but got used to it.

I came in at tea-time, went straight into the dining hall. My son went straight off. Knew nobody. Felt all up to here [her throat] but got over it. The hardest thing was being waited on – led to the table, toilet and bedroom [she is blind]. I'm very independent and I like to do things for myself. They are kind and I ought to be grateful. I've got a placid nature – always done things for myself, I don't know other people's feelings – the different things people have to endure . . . The most difficult thing is not being able to go out for walks on my own. I miss the outdoors and gardening. I used to be up at eight and get the housework done by ten so that I could get out in the garden.

I miss my garden, had two nice lawns, grew rose trees [and she talked about a busy life with clubs and meetings, making 800 Easter cakes for a sale, and how she had wanted to cut herself off from all these things on coming into The Pines].

I came in an ambulance, was car-sick. I was shown my room, had one by myself to start with. It was difficult but I had been in hospital before. The people were most difficult to get used to – all were very friendly. At home it is quiet, no next-door neighbour. I lived next to the farm, I missed the noises of that for getting up, the cows going for milking.

Matron came and greeted me. I thought it was all very nice. I couldn't sleep for two or three nights. It was better than I thought. I remembered the old workhouse.

It is apparent that some residents arrived close to a meal-time and therefore went along to the dining hall soon after arrival. One had enjoyed this because she was 'kept in conversation'. However, it may well be difficult as an early experience for many people. A similar point is made in a recent review of residential care (Personal Social Services Council, 1977): 'Above all, he should not be led into a full sitting room and left to cope on his own.'

Two people talked about feeling lonely or not sleeping at night and staff comments on how this could be altered are discussed later. The essential part is to separate the aspects that cannot be modified – missing the noises of the farm – from those that could be handled differently, such as information about possessions.

The admission process appeared to me a crucial and neglected part of the way residents learnt to behave in a new setting. In the report which I produced for staff I drew attention to some points.

Several interesting things emerge:

(1) Residents often said they couldn't remember what happened when they came in. But when I asked who brought them and whom they met from the home they remembered a lot. In particular they remembered talking to a senior staff member, going to their rooms, going into the sitting room and their first meal. Therefore what happens on the first day is very important.

(2) The difficulty of being in a strange place at night-time. Loneliness and strangeness are most apparent then. For some residents the nights remain times of loneliness and pain.

(3) The little residents remember of anyone talking about what they could bring into the home. They had been told they could bring in a commode but others had left behind ornaments that they wished they had brought with them.

Some had been able to collect these later; in other cases they had gone. 'I wonder what happened to my radio. I'd like that now' said someone. The concern about doing the right thing was so great that many people never brought in things they wished they had.

(4) From my observation of the admission of a holiday visitor: he arrived with the social worker, had a brief discussion with a senior staff member outside the office, was shown up to his room. Meanwhile the social worker came into the office, handed over his pension book, talked to staff members, said that he wanted his pocket money but would spend it if he had it. She left. Later a care attendant came into the office: 'I've unpacked his case and brought down these tablets.' What struck me was that initiative or responsibility was taken away at so early a stage. First, the social worker dominated the early discussion outside the office, she handed in his pension book, she said 'perhaps he shouldn't have his money'; the care attendant brought down the tablets.

To me this is an important example of the way responsibility is removed from residents. I believe incidents like this admission process are part of the reason for the apathy that nearly everyone seems to dislike. The comment of one of the residents – 'I took it as it came, resigned to doing what was expected of me' – is an example of what people expect to find.

(5) Those residents who were most satisfied were usually those who thought they had played a major part in making the decision to come in.

(6) The important point is that the first impressions lead on to fixed attitudes. In the example above other people (the social worker and staff) decided what would happen to the new resident – and so a resident gets used to a situation where other people make decisions for him.

Social workers who accompanied old people into residential homes were aware of the way the group of residents dominated proceedings at an early stage. They would tell a new resident not to put a bag down on a particular chair: 'That won't be her chair, she won't be sitting there.' Similarly an individual's picture of life in the home would vary according to which sitting area she went to. People had had very different experiences in one sitting area on holiday and then in a different sitting area next time they came in.

Staff felt that it was important to be hospitable to the new resident, and it is apparent from several comments that senior staff members succeeded in conveying their interest. 'Matron came and greeted me', more than one resident said. Some staff members suggested that taking a case and unpacking it is the sort of hospitality that one would show to a guest. 'How else do you show that they are welcome?' asked someone.

Nevertheless, the example of the holiday visitor illustrates a type of hospitality that leads to dependence. There is no reason why an admission scheme should not foster independence and convey warmth, if that is what is desired. Other examples of socialisation into set patterns of behaviour, for instance, keeping the room tidy, will be discussed later.

# Chapter 6

---

# DAILY LIFE FOR RESIDENTS IN
# THE PINES

The style of life of residents at The Pines is portrayed in this chapter through the eyes of myself as participant observer and of residents. A comparison can be made with the staff view in Chapter 9. Both the staff's and residents' viewpoints will have similarities to and differences from other establishments.

It is difficult to capture the key elements of life in a residential home. Discussing this problem, a geriatrician referred to trace elements in plants – elements which are present only in minute quantities, are difficult to analyse but are essential to the well-being of the plant. Hopefully some of these trace elements that make up the sound, sight, smell and feel of life at The Pines are captured in what follows.

### A TYPICAL DAY

About 6.30 a.m. residents who will need a lot of help with dressing are woken up. The remainder will hear a knock on their door between 6.45 and 7.00 and the care assistant will bring in a cup of tea. Some residents are already awake – 'You're late this morning'; others slowly wake up. At 7.30 the care assistant does a second round and collects up the cups. One man says he doesn't feel well enough to get up. A woman asks for her red and black dress from the sewing room. Somebody else wants another blanket.

There is a bit more noise and bustle. Some people are sitting waiting to be helped with the next stage of dressing; others are persuaded to start getting up. One resident who has become highly dependent is left sleeping in her room.

8.00: Some residents move downstairs and sit in a sitting area till breakfast. Others go straight to the tables. The vacuum cleaner is going – 'We have to get used to that music' says a resident. There is a succession of greetings between staff and residents as different people meet. Residents greet each other more quietly.

The corridor from the lift is crowded with slow-moving residents, with sticks, zimmer frames and an occasional wheelchair.

8.30: Breakfast. Everyone is seated. The senior staff are behind the hatch serving the food; the assistants take it to the residents. Cereal or grapefruit, bread or toast, poached egg and baked beans. The residents are sitting four to a table; cutlery and china are standard, so are serviettes but each ring is marked with a name; there are cloths on the table. There is a teapot on each table and the group has usually decided who is going to pour. The meal is fairly quiet. Second helpings are taken round for those who want them. The clatter of dishes being washed up is heard. Some residents get up to go; others finish off their meal, talk, or wait for tablets which are taken round at the end of the meal. Some people have ordered a daily paper and these are handed round.

9.00: The residents make their way to the sitting rooms, some with staff assistance. One or two help others by collecting sticks or walking frames. A blind woman is seen to her room by a resident. Two or three residents go into the kitchen to finish the last of the drying-up. Most of the residents go to their particular places in the sitting areas. One or two in each room read the paper; some are already dozing; others will knit, sew, or chat.

10.30: The drinks trolley is taken round. Most residents stick to their regular drinks, milky coffee, coffee cooled with cold water, or squash. A lot of chatter between the assistant and the residents, about last night's TV programme, children at home, relatives' visits. One or two residents have been in their bedrooms, coming out when they hear the drinks come round.

Meanwhile some residents are being bathed – by two assistants if they are very heavy or frail, otherwise by one.

Letters are brought round by the secretary. One resident gets up to lay the tables for lunch; someone else has walked down to the town to place his daily bet. A woman calls in to see her father before she collects her children from school.

11.00: Bathing continues. Residents see a senior staff member as she goes to each sitting area in turn – 'What do you think about those tablets I have been given?'; 'How are you getting on with the plans for the coffee morning?'; 'Do you know if I am going out for the day on Sunday?' – she is asked.

Two people go to the nearby pub for a drink.

12.00: A start is made towards getting some residents ready for lunch. They are taken to the toilet or helped along to the dining hall. The more fit leave it until later to make a move.

12.30: Nearly everyone is sitting at the tables. Two are missing – one man is always late, but an assistant goes to look for the other person. It is a noisier meal than breakfast. Meals are served up at the hatch and carried round. A few people need their food cut up; someone doesn't like what she has got. A man gets up to go to the toilet. The second course is served. A similar pattern to breakfast – some wait for tablets, others leave, one or two dry the glasses.

1.00: Many have settled back in their armchairs. Several have gone to their bedrooms to lie down. The TV is on in one sitting room.

2.00: The afternoon is more leisurely than the morning. Cleaners have finished their work. Some people are bathed; others doze or listen to the radio. There are more visitors and more residents go out – to clubs or for a walk. Two people read books, several knit.

2.30: Tea is brought round on a trolley. The TV is put on in the men's sitting room for the racing.

5.00: High tea. The pattern is similar to other meals. There is a cooked main course followed by cakes and bread and butter.

6.15: Eight residents have met in the dining hall to play bingo. One of them calls the numbers. Later, a staff member takes over for a short time; the residents are glad when a visitor offers to call the numbers. Around the rest of the home the televisions are all on. There are more visitors. One or two people are bathed before bed.

7.15: An evening drinks trolley is taken round with a selection of hot milk drinks, squash and biscuits. Those who need help in getting to bed are taken to their rooms by the care assistants. Several others choose to go to bed soon after 8.00.

9.00: Most residents are in bed. Four of those who are still up gather in a sitting room near the office to chat and watch TV. Some men have stayed in their own sitting room upstairs. One man has been across to the pub.

10.00: Those who are downstairs have a cup of tea with staff. One by one they go to bed.

11.00: All residents are in their rooms. Some have had sleeping tablets. One or two may need to call staff during the night for help to get to the toilet.

### CONTROL OF LIFE-STYLE

The key questions which are examined in this section are: 'How far is a resident able to decide how she will live?'; 'what factors exert influence on her life-style?'. The items selected as indicators (see above, pp. 32–3) are used as headings for this discussion.

(1) *Money*

All residents were expected to hand over their pension books to the secretary. She made arrangements to cash their weekly pension, would deduct the payment due to the local authority and distributed the remainder every Friday to residents in the sitting rooms. This was termed 'pocket money'. Residents might keep all or part of this money, together with any other they might have. If they wished they could deposit money in the office for safe keeping. There was a notice in the wardrobe in each room stating that the local authority would take no responsibility for money missing from rooms.

Not all residents meekly submitted.

I was in the office when a hunchbacked, determined woman came in as a resident. The secretary asked her for her pension book so that she could change the designated post office, and also so that the matron would be granted authorisation to cash the pension. The resident would not hear of it. 'I won't sign anything; I'm going home soon' she said. 'She knows her own mind too well. You can't pull the wool over her eyes' said a senior staff member.

Another resident had to pay more than the minimum because of her assets. She did not like being at the home and found herself persuaded to stay there. Her anxiety about what was happening to her made her determined and she refused to pay anything except through her solicitor. Her solicitor was informed and he paid the bill. Later it transpired she had had enough money in her handbag to pay the bill. She had not been asked to give up her handbag, though staff suspected she might have had the money.

At any one period there were about three residents who were given no money because they were regarded as too confused and the money would then be placed in an account for them. If they were thought to need items such as toiletries or clothing it would be spent for them. It was assumed that residents did not understand what was going on. However, one resident commented: 'They used to keep my money in the office and buy me clothes, stockings and that', so she had been aware that her money was spent for her.

Some residents appeared to give most of the sum they had left (about £3) to their relatives. Staff would feel considerable anger towards such relatives, especially when they were thought to visit only to get the money. One man had a daughter who handled all his money and gave him what she considered he needed. He was left with very little. One day he told me how he had asked her for another pair of shoes. 'You've got a pair of shoes in your room', she replied, 'you don't need another.' 'I do really though', he added to me, 'because I keep doing wee on my shoes.' A woman was unable to pay to go out on outings or for a drink because she was left with so little.

On the other hand, residents who had few relatives and spent little might save a lot of money. One man had to be taken to hospital from the home. When he was about to go he handed over £516 which he had saved under his mattress. Had staff known about it, they would have banked it and this would have increased his capital to the point where he would have had to pay a larger contribution. The resident was as well aware of this as the staff. There were other occasions when staff found themselves with information about additional finances that residents had not declared. Staff felt torn between loyalty to the resident and to the local authority.

### (2) Cleaning

Domestic workers were employed to clean the home. Expenditure cuts had meant these staff were employed for fewer hours so areas like the dining hall were polished less often. The significant factor here is that the bedrooms were cleaned each morning by domestic staff and residents were expected to keep out of their rooms until they were cleaned.

Care assistants made the beds. A few residents made their own, though some thought this was not allowed. No resident did any washing or ironing, though a few relatives did take clothes away to wash at home.

Several points emerged through considering this area. The domestic staff might grumble about rooms which they considered too untidy. Mrs Draxton moved into a single room. 'It was the first morning I was in my new room. I hadn't had time to get straight. My arm ached appalling. She [a domestic] came in – "I'm not having this room like this" she said. So this morning I got up and tried to get it tidy. "That's better, my dear" she said to me.' Another time Mrs Draxton was in trouble for leaving some clothes out on her bed and not putting them away in drawers.

There was no consultation with residents about how often they liked the room cleaned or how they liked it done. There seemed no encouragement to residents to consider doing it for themselves, in fact no joint planning about what was needed. This is significant in view of the fact that a survey of isolated elderly by Tunstall (1966) showed that cleaning was second only to cooking as the task carried out by most people at least once per week.

### (3) Clothing

Residents had separate wardrobes and chests of drawers. Some clothes would be kept in these, some centrally in the linen room. Certain residents had more clothes kept centrally, but it was not possible to be certain whether these were the more confused residents (the stated reason) or the more passive ones. It is easier to keep clothes centrally than to distribute them around.

While the stated policy was that residents could change clothes whenever they wanted, some residents were said to abuse this. 'Could I have my red and black dress? I don't know where it is, it has been taken away' said Mrs Hughes. 'Yes, some of the summer ones were put away' was the reply from the care assistant, 'I'll see and come back if I can.' To me she added: 'I shan't do anything. We took her clothes away a few weeks ago because she kept changing them and putting them to the wash.' The effect of this type of deception could only be to disorient further someone who was already thought to be confused.

The general pattern was that residents could wear what they wanted and keep control of it. There were difficulties about sorting clothes – one man regularly confided that he was wearing someone else's pants – but while this was sometimes correct and partly accounted for by poor marking of clothes, there were times when he was mistaken. The standard of washing and ironing was high, though staff accepted there were occasional mistakes in sorting clothes.

Residents dressed differently and mostly chose what they wanted to wear. The control of staff was shown by their ability to control the quality of the service. While nearly all residents smelt fresh, Mr Gasden's clothes were not washed frequently enough and regularly he smelt of urine.

Two other incidents stand out. The first was a comment from a relative that her father had found it difficult to get used to life in the home 'because even on his own he used to like pottering around. He liked it a bit scruffy – in the home it was too clean, but *he eventually got used to a collar and tie*, etc.' This shows the way expectations become introduced. I had not picked up any mention that men had to wear ties; presumably this expectation was passed on to new residents and all the men ended up wearing ties. In the second incident two care assistants decided to snip a bit of lace off someone's nightdress ('she'll never notice') because they wanted it for a lavender bag to sell at a coffee morning to raise funds for the residents: an example of priorities getting so mixed up that an act of mild delinquency takes place.

(4)  *Daily programme*
Residents were free to plan a large part of their day. However, this simple statement masks some of the more subtle influences. Residents were not allowed to stay in bed. There was anxiety amongst staff that once one person did that, everyone would want to. A senior staff member said: 'The doctor says Mrs Black needs to rest more. We'll put her to bed in the afternoons, perhaps that will help. Her niece was here and said "Couldn't she stay in bed, she'd be in bed at home". It is difficult to know when it's best to let them lie, sometimes it's not in their best interests. But she is 92 and I think she'd probably have got over it more quickly if she'd stayed in bed.'

Miss Johns, usually very compliant, said 'Sometimes I wish I could stay in bed longer', and others felt like her. Mrs Sidney was grateful that staff had persuaded her to get up when she felt depressed. 'You get so used to the routine. You are better for getting up. I don't mind getting up now' she said. Mrs Pinker, who was blind, was one of several who got up before being called.

I'm happy about getting up; I woke about three-thirty a.m. yesterday and didn't sleep again. Got out and cleaned my teeth, tidied my drawer, back into bed and do some knitting. It passes the time – well I shouldn't wish the time away, mustn't say 'Oh I wish the day was over', it's wrong to wish that. I ought to like the day though, if I'm well and happy. If I was in pain or desperate I might feel different.

I would get up at the time we do anyway. I start getting dressed and washed. Get up about seven-twenty and I'm ready by eight o'clock, it could be before that.

She went on to describe the rest of her day.

Miss Johns comes and picks me up. I listen to the radio. Always have something at breakfast – the only trouble is that the toast isn't crisp, all steamy, doughy. Love to get to the dining hall and hear all the conversations.

Then I go to the sitting room. Mostly knitting or talking, someone might read the paper to me. I like to hear people talking but I'm not used to talking to other people, not a conversationalist.

You get a lot of fun from listening. You shut your eyes and listen, you'd be surprised what you hear. I knit on and off all day.

Come in my room from dinner-time till half-past three, listen to my book, snooze, listen to the radio. The doctor says 'You should lay on your bed, it's advisable to rest'. I go back to the sitting room and knit, more knitting.

Come to bed about eight o'clock. Some of the TV is confusing. I miss a lot. I like coming in to my room at night, being quiet, I don't get bored.

Mrs Pinker loved going to meals to hear all the bustle. When they were in the home, residents were usually expected to go in to meals. This served as a check on people's whereabouts and their eating habits.

Mrs Knight was well aware of staff expectations: 'I feel ill when I get up. Don't know how I get down to meals. They like you to go down if you can.'

Miss Manfield didn't mind getting up, but added: 'I get short of breath. Sometimes I don't care if I go to breakfast – I feel faint sometimes. Do you have to go to breakfast?'

There was some uncertainty about use of bedrooms. The problem was that domestics had to get in to clean rooms. Interpretations of what this meant varied. Senior staff members said that residents should be out while their rooms were cleaned; the norm appeared to be 'do not use bedrooms until 12 noon', while some residents genuinely thought they were not meant to go in their rooms at any time of the day.

Care assistants or domestic staff, anxious to get on with their work, might tell residents they were not meant to be in their rooms. Interestingly it was accepted that two residents did spend all day in their rooms. They were regarded as eccentric or stubborn and the cleaning went on round them. This is an illustration of the way in which stubbornness can lead to an individual modification of norms. It shows the importance for the elderly of asserting mastery – and that it is necessary to find socially acceptable ways of this happening.

With some other provisos, residents were free to plan their day. Visitors could come and go without making appointments; residents were free to go shopping, wander round the grounds or the town. Inevitably for many the constraints were to do with their own limited ability – there were variations from the fully mobile, to those walking short distances with zimmer frames, to people who needed staff assistance for any movement. Even given these increased dependencies, some chose to go out to clubs (when transport was arranged) while others did not.

Miss Carpenter liked to keep active and, though she needed a stick, was more active than most residents. She was glad of transport to take her to Red Cross meetings.

I look forward to the Sunday service, Gospel meetings, holidays and Red Cross. I like doing things for people, help Miss X down in the lift, wash up. I have tablets to take when I wake at about five in the morning. Get myself dressed – hope I always shall. I sit down in the lounge after breakfast – talk – sometimes go in and see Mrs Y. After lunch I read in my bedroom from about three-fifteen to four-fifteen. Sometimes there are entertainments or I watch TV. Two of the others decide what goes on.

It has already been mentioned that fit residents could go to bed when they wished. Those needing staff help had to be got ready earlier, and indeed got up in the morning earlier.

Mr Peat described his evening. 'After tea we watch TV – we all like the same sorts of things – go to bed about ten or ten-thirty.'

Mrs Smith similarly watched TV and then went to bed about eight-thirty. 'I don't want to stay up any longer and then I read in bed.'

Several residents described parts of the day that seemed boring. Some, like Mrs Knight, found physical handicap limited what they could do.

I don't like getting up because I can't stand long. Don't eat much breakfast. I make my bed myself. They know if I leave it that I can't manage it. I sit in the bedroom after breakfast – quiet till ten-thirty – I can't sew or knit. I read books in the morning. I don't talk a lot, like being quiet. I don't look forward to meals much. The doctor just says 'That's your old stomach complaint'. After lunch I have to sit quiet till half-past three, have to rest my legs which swell.

In spite of handicap she said that she didn't get bored.

Mrs Tanner clearly missed the activity of family life. She seemed happiest when there were things to do.

I used to get up at seven-thirty – the whole family did – grand-daughter used to say 'Not coming down early again!'. I wouldn't get up quite so early now if I could choose; I just take a few minutes to get dressed and then I go straight down to breakfast. I strip my bed before breakfast and then make it, I don't like anyone else making my bed; it takes about fifteen minutes. I'm out of the room by nine-thirty. I read, but can't read all the time. Read the paper – then it's coffee. 'What, eleven o'clock already?' I think. The morning doesn't seem long.

Afternoons seem endless. Worse than the morning. Go out when it's nicer. Sometimes when I go out with my grand-daughter I walk home – up to the railway line – or go to the shops with her. Have visitors quite frequently, once or twice a week. In the evenings they have TV, silly programmes. I don't like westerns. I go to bed at nine o'clock. I used to stay up and watch the programmes but I'd be the only one. I like watching *Mastermind*, I like things like that that have some reality. Don't talk much, they don't like it. They're a dumb league in the afternoon. Don't play bingo because I can't see to play.

Staff were uncertain as to how far residents should be left when sitting passively. There were occasional attempts to interest them – one staff member tried to interest a resident in some magazines. Another would turn on the TV for residents – on one occasion when she left a resident said: 'Good, now we can turn it off; she always puts it on, though we don't want it.' Sometimes staff members tried to persuade residents to go out for a drink or do a puzzle. Mr Peters muttered to me that he didn't like doing puzzles but, perversely, seemed to get pleasure from having completed one.

Staff were also concerned to keep residents mobile. Residents had different opinions about how appropriate this was. Mrs Pinker described a very old resident, Mrs White, who was being made to walk. Someone who sat at her table thought it hard to keep pressing her. Mrs Pinker said: 'I think if you give up you'd give up for ever. If I thought I wouldn't do any knitting I could sit and mope.'

The tensions were focused most clearly when there were 'events' on. Although starting from a belief that residents were free to decide, pressures were often exerted on residents to attend, both for the sake of the 'performer' as well as from a belief that it would be good for the resident.

Mrs Quigley, Mrs Sidney and Miss Carpenter discussed the pending visit of someone who was coming to show them how to make Christmas decorations. Mrs Quigley: 'I think I'll go up to my room now. I don't want to go to that group this week.' Miss Carpenter: 'I don't want to go. I can't do anything with my hands.' Mrs Sidney: 'I shan't go either.' Before Mrs Quigley had left a senior staff member came in. 'Are you coming, Mrs Quigley?' 'Oh, all right then.' Miss Carpenter added: 'Well, I could just sit and watch.' Mrs Sidney chimed in 'I may have visitors', and she was very glad later to have a visitor and consequently a legitimate excuse.

It seemed at times that the church services in the home were boosted by the presence of the confused and the passive who would go along when directed.

## (5) Bathing

Residents were bathed once a week. A record was kept of the date and comments were added about soreness or need for a chiropodist.

Most residents had got used to being bathed by other people, either relatives or district nurses, before coming into the home. The few who were embarrassed at the experience soon got used to it, helped by the staff attitude. Mrs White said: 'I'm used to it now though it was embarrassing. I know the girls. It's lovely to have a nice drop of water. A good many people never knew what it was like to have a bath.'

Nearly everybody was grateful for the help. Mrs Roberts, a large woman, who was often bathed by two staff, found that 'they jabbered to each other about their husbands'. She much preferred being bathed by one person. One day when I helped bath somebody I found similarly that the care assistant and I were talking to each other and the resident was being ignored.

While residents were glad to be helped they were often resentful about the timing. In spite of listening for cues – 'I wonder if it will be my turn soon. Mrs Smith has had another bath since I have' – residents were often taken by surprise and did not like suddenly having to go off for a bath.

Mrs Richardson: 'It's my turn for a bath soon. I just said to my friend that I didn't really want one, not today. Still you can't tell them that. I'll feel better after I've had it. I don't like it when they bath me at twelve. That's too much of a rush before lunch. I thought they might do that today. Still I must be thankful they didn't bath me then.'

Mrs Sidney felt that 'you can't be too long because someone else needs to be helped'.

Mrs Smith said about another occasion: 'I never have got annoyed, only once. That was the other day. They came and took me for a bath in the evening. I prefer to be advised when, I had some visitors coming. I wouldn't say "no" but it is annoying.' This was in marked contrast with situations where staff took note of residents' feelings about times of bathing or gave some advance warning. 'All right for a bath in half an hour, Mr Gasden?'

One day when Mrs Williams had a bad cold she didn't think she should have a bath. The senior staff member thought she should. 'I've got to go and have a bath. I don't want to, still I suppose I've got to, got to obey orders.'

There was a firmness to the policy about bathing. Holiday visitors were bathed even when they protested that they had had a bath just before coming in.

It is, of course, unusual for most people to bath during the day. A large part of the stress for the residents was that they had to undress and dress again, a procedure that was often tiring. This raises the question as to whether changes in staffing hours or of times when residents get up would alleviate this.

## (6)  *Food*

At breakfast and tea, teapots, bread and butter and jam were placed on the table. The remainder of the meal was served on to plates in the kitchen and the care assistants took the meals to residents. They had a good knowledge of likes and dislikes ('Mrs Sidney won't have any gravy') but residents were dependent on the memory and concern of staff. Some residents were prepared to ask for a meal to be changed – 'I don't really want any potato today' – but most accepted what they were given. Some would add: 'It's not quite what I wanted, but I'll have it.'

The quality of the food was excellent and there was usually a choice of main course. Residents commented on how much they enjoyed it. Mr Murphy said: 'I enjoy the meals – too much, though. It's good and well cooked. They can't cook it how you would like it, though. Everything is cooked soft. I was more used to food in bigger lumps, pork chops and things.' Inevitably it was different from what people were used to (there was more or less salt) and the difficulty of adjusting to this highlights the significance of food. Food seems the symbol of the intimacy of their past life and at least as significant to men as to women.

The fact of being waited on by staff is also important. Restaurants and hotels are the situations when we expect to be waited on, and there is a strange duality in this relationship. The customer has the power to select what he requires but also feels very dependent. 'Shall I ask for more milk?' 'Will the waiter be surly or pleasant?' 'We have waited here for hours.' 'Shh, dear, don't make a fuss.' Those comments reflect some of the uncertainty. In the old age home the power of the customer is reduced (he is not paying a bill in the same way), while that of the person serving seems greatly increased. The care assistant has knowledge of most of a resident's life and considerable power in other spheres of living. It is not so easy to assert yourself. Early in my research notes I described this as 'the powerlessness of the hotel guest'.

In fact there was little formal pressure on residents to eat particular foods. They could eat just vegetables or no vegetables at all. Yet there was a reluctance to leave residents with their choices. 'I should have a bit of meat' said a care assistant. At its extreme this could lead to feeding by staff.

Mr Page came in to lunch. He looked dishevelled and was not well. He had brought a bottle of beer in with him. He was deaf and often would not use a hearing aid, which made little difference. Staff poured out his beer for him; he turned down any food. The care assistant put his bib on him and tried to push the food in. 'You must have something, it's good for you.' Most of it dribbled down his chin. Later another care assistant tried: 'Matron says you have got to have this sweet.' He pushed it away: 'I'll have it for tea.' There was a discussion between staff and residents. 'He needs his food, he'll get weak without it . . .'

I was surprised on my first day at the large helpings of food eaten by residents and even more surprised to see residents consuming second helpings of the first course. Clearly I was wrong to have assumed that the old would eat less. There was another side, however. 'Matron likes to see you eat a lot' said Mrs Smith.

An example:

SENIOR STAFF MEMBER TO MRS ROBERTS: 'You'll have some more custard and apple. Here Mr Clough, give it to her.'

MRS ROBERTS: 'No, thank you.'

STAFF MEMBER: 'Yes she will, put it down.'

ME: 'Would you?'

MRS ROBERTS: 'Not really.'

STAFF MEMBER: 'Go on, put it there, she'll have it.'

Mrs Roberts had pushed her plate away, but said reluctantly: 'Well, I'll see what I can do.' Presumably it is very satisfying for staff to see residents enjoying their food.

Timing of attendance at meals is also a visible reminder of one's status. Mrs Williams disliked waiting before a meal. 'It's like school-children; still you've got to put those things aside.' It was noticeable that the fittest came last to meals. Residents attached importance to getting to meals on time. Meals were served at set times: 8.30 a.m., 12.30 p.m. and 5.00 p.m. 'I'm afraid for my life of being late' said

Miss Brinton. 'I don't think I'd get any if I came late, though people are excused.' Other residents expressed similar anxieties.

There was an expectation that residents would come in to meals if they were in the home. Recognised illness was a legitimate excuse; the visit of a relative was grudgingly accepted. Otherwise people were persuaded to come in and 'just sit', or 'just eat a little'. Meal-times provided a check on the whereabouts of residents. Provided they had stated they were going out, residents were perfectly free to miss meals.

Another aspect of the method of serving was that there were frequent shouts across the dining hall – 'Gravy, Mrs Sidney?' – especially to certain residents who were more assertive. By contrast one care assistant would go round the table in advance asking what was wanted. 'I do like to be asked, not just have a meal put down' said Mrs Tanner.

Having served the meal, staff appeared to stand round like vultures waiting to pounce on empty plates. Residents must have felt the rush and few stayed chatting at the end of the meal.

It is easy to forget that the freedom to manage life-style is not constrained only by staff. It is constrained also by other residents. I had been prepared for worse table manners than I saw. In spite of the fact that behaviour was nearer normal than I had expected, bad table manners were mentioned by residents most often as the most annoying behaviour of others. There were comments like 'I shouldn't want to eat at some tables'; 'table habits are annoying'; 'Mr Page coughs at the table'; 'I have to tell them not to do some things'. The extreme situation was rare – a member of staff described a meal when one man said he couldn't sit and watch another eat, while a different man was spitting away.

Residents would exert direct control on behaviour. Mrs Richardson described such an event: 'I went to pour a second cup of tea one evening and he said "You are in a temper". I said "Indeed not, don't say that about me". No one must touch the teapot when he is about. He is ninety-two years of age and he shakes some tea in the saucer sometimes.'

But meals provided positive stimulation also: 'I love to get down to the dining hall and hear all the conversations'; 'there's something nice about going down to meals – you all meet together again and the attendants are ready to serve us'; 'I enjoy meals, hearing what everybody is saying', said three residents.

## (7) *Medical services*

Residents were able to choose their own doctor. This was important to them. The procedure was that if they felt ill or wished to see the doctor they would ask the staff to make arrangements. This gave staff some power of interpretation as to whether a doctor was needed or not. Mrs Williams used to get her son to take her out to the doctor's surgery because 'I get the feeling they [the staff] think I'm making a fuss'. She was the only person who went out to see a doctor.

There were other examples of the constraints imposed by this system. In the first a senior staff member decided that it was not necessary to call the doctor for two residents who had asked to see him; in the second, about a different resident, Mrs Sidney stated: 'They should have called the doctor days ago.'

The doctor usually saw the patient in a bedroom, though there were a few occasions when doctors carried out a consultation in a sitting room with other residents around.

The regulations of the local authority stated that all medicines and drugs were to be kept by the staff unless a doctor specified otherwise. In fact all drugs were held centrally and distributed at the end of meals, though a few residents did buy occasional cough sweets or Aspro. This meant that residents did not keep their own drugs.

Medicines themselves exerted a considerable control over life-style, both beneficial and harmful. The beneficial aspect was in alleviating pain and controlling chronic conditions; the harmful side was that, in spite of attempts by staff and occasionally by doctors, there was a general agreement that residents ended up with too many tablets, and this might lead to the residents' confusion. Some staff felt that sometimes antibiotics were used inappropriately and led to a slower, more painful death. Residents were often uncertain about the value of their medication. Mr Jepson complained about the tablets he was taking: 'It's not worth having them if they make you feel so rotten. I'd rather die.'

## (8)  Furniture and decorating

Residents were allowed to take in small possessions, including a chair and commode. There was little room for anything else and no opportunity to store the furniture of the home. The position of the bed, central with access on both sides, made for convenience in making beds. Many people in bed-sitters would have a bed against the walls where it functions more like a couch. Most rooms had only a few bits and pieces around. There was little that made a permanent feeling of possession, for example, pictures hung on the walls. People were allowed to carpet their bedrooms but the carpet had to stay when a resident left or died. No resident had had her room painted or decorated to suit her own taste.

The personality of the resident would influence the amount of control that was exerted on her to keep the room tidy. Some rooms on the ground floor were passed by all visitors coming into the home and there seemed greater pressure for these to be kept tidy. A determined resident would be able to have a lot of clutter around.

In each room there was a small drawer with a lock in the bedside cupboard. The keys of some of these had been lost, leaving some people with nowhere to lock anything up. The request of one man to fit a lock to his wardrobe was turned down by a senior staff member.

It has already been noted that residents were not supposed to be in their rooms at certain times.

These indicators of resident control proved useful. While their links to the typology of homes will not be made until Chapter 11, the indicators allow comparison with other styles of living.

### NEEDS AND RESOURCES

Let us take the case of a resident who was living in her own house prior to admission. There would be limitations also on her ability to control her life-style in areas discussed above (bathing, cleaning, etc.). It would be necessary to take account of her resources – health, money, housing, access to support. Thus she might be too handicapped to cook a meal and consequently dependent on someone cooking for her. Similar examples could be multiplied in relation to any of the other headings.

The significant difference between the two life-styles is that in the old age home resources are made available to meet needs. However, the more resources a resident needs, the more she is likely to lose control of the manner in which those resources should be provided. Gubrium suggests that satisfaction is dependent on a balance between activity resources and activity norms. Therefore if an individual has the resources available to match the expectations of the immediate society in which she lives (including her own expectations) then she can be said to be coping.

Transfer to a residential home profoundly alters the balance between resources and norms. The resources side of the equation receives a sudden boost. The individual is freed from some of the anxieties of daily living – paying bills, keeping the house warm – and receives help with meeting personal needs – bathing and feeding. Consequently she has more time, and may be in better health, to do other things. But at the same time the other side of the equation, the norms or the expectations of those around her, also alter. The past balance goes haywire and a new harmony needs to be established. It is crucial to realise that there are positives for the resident through the provision of additional resources; yet, grateful as residents may be for those resources, in situations where they have minimal control over the way the resource is provided they are often uneasy.

### PUBLIC AND PRIVATE

It is difficult to capture the key elements of life in an old age institution. A comparison with other styles of living is helpful. The normal pattern of living in society is to live on one's own or in a small group. This group is more or less secluded from the rest of the community and there are clear boundaries between the group and the outside. Inside the individuals eat, sleep, relax. They emerge when they wish to meet other people, go to work, play, or for any other reason; similarly they may invite others into their base. One of the essential changes for an individual in an old age institution is that the privacy of the base is lost.

This is of fundamental importance. Between the inside and outside of one's own home is a clear boundary, however often it may be crossed. Is the resident to see the base as her own room, or the whole institution? The first is too small and, in this establishment at least, not a private living base; the latter is too large, too public and too diffuse. Mrs Pinker had lived in the country before admission. She had lived in a row of houses and would stop and speak to people. She never had anyone into her house and never went into another house. In a way she thought she lost contact with the outside world. But within her house she had been very happy with her husband and children, and her whole life had centred on them and her garden. It was hard for her to transfer to a situation where there was no clear inside base and outside world.

It may be possible to make the individual's room in the old age home approximate more closely to this idea of a base. At The Pines there were severe limitations. Staff would enter rooms without knocking except for the very first call of the day. They would go into cupboards to take out or put clothes away; the cleaners would similarly go in when they needed to. When Mr Fothergill thought he was losing things he asked whether he might have a lock on his wardrobe. A senior staff member thought this highly inappropriate. 'What would the staff think if the residents began to lock things up? They would imagine they were not trusted.' Perhaps to begin to serve the function of a base residents would need to be able to lock the doors of the rooms.

An additional factor in the different living-styles concerns use of bedrooms. It has already been noted that residents were expected not to use the rooms until the cleaners had finished. However, some residents believed they were not supposed to use the rooms at any time. Others clearly felt that staff wanted them to come out and sit in the sitting rooms. Two residents did use their rooms as their regular base (they achieved this by ignoring the cajoling and persuading of staff). The rest used the sitting room as the normal living place and their rooms more as a bolt-hole, when they wanted a sleep or to receive visitors.

The result was that most people lived their lives in public in a way

they never had before (a few had experienced far more public living –
in the army or other institutions). They would sit and read, or knit,
or chat, or doze alongside other people. These experiences are shared
usually only in one's intimate living group. Here they were shared with
people they had not selected as friends.

Lipman (1968) comes to similar conclusions:

> Before field studies started it was assumed that the residents' bed-
> rooms would be venues for receiving fellow residents, that the
> designation 'bed-sitting room' given by the Ministry of Health ...
> indicated that some social life would take place in the bedrooms
> ... social life in the homes took place almost exclusively in the
> sitting rooms, and, to a lesser extent, in the dining rooms. The
> sitting rooms were the centres, the cockpits of social life in the Homes.

It is in this context, he argues, that it is necessary to consider the
way individuals develop 'rights' to particular chairs and places. 'It
seems that a person regularly occupying a chair exercises his authority
to exist as a social entity – his identity – in a physical location ... In
other words, the chair becomes a symbol of the occupant's social
existence ...'

In The Pines, as in many other old age institutions, residents did
exercise rights to particular chairs. Clearly this was linked to the fact
that the sitting room was the centre of social life but it is also linked
to the uncertainty about one's base.

Two further points make this uncertainty even more significant. The
first is the style of sitting rooms in the home. Since they were open-
plan with one side open to the corridor, living in the sitting room
meant that one was also living in a corridor. Thus people passing by
had to be greeted and acknowledged and might drop in for a chat.
Secondly, since the tasks of daily living were being carried out by the
staff, the resident had more time than ever before for 'non-work' activity.
Consequently, instead of living in comparative seclusion and emerging to
meet friends or to shop, the pattern for residents was to live in a semi-
public group and to retreat when separateness was wanted.

Therefore boundaries did not have the same significance. Nor were
residents protected by the boundary in the same way. Playing host to
friends means inviting them to cross into one's base, but at The Pines
friends would come in uninvited. The resident was no longer able to play
host, nor to refuse to see unwelcome visitors. So the very freedom of
visitors to drop in when they wished and without letting staff know,
a freedom that was positively welcomed by most residents, created
further changes in living-style. It would be difficult to find ways of
fulfilling the role of host or of protecting the resident.

At The Pines the visitor assumed most of the power that normally
belongs to the host. Many visitors chose to talk to their friend or

relative in the sitting room. Often there was no spare chair on which they might sit. The fact that they were standing heightened the passivity of the old person, and it was often the visitor who initiated conversation with others in the room. The role of the host in receiving, settling and providing for the visitor largely disappeared.

Occasional comments point to the fact that visitors, usually other people's, could be intrusive. Mrs Sidney commented that she would go somewhere else when this happened. Most visitors had a specific purpose, that of visiting a particular resident. There was little need for protection from these. On the other hand intrusions from staff, other residents, or interested people were not so easy to handle.

I was aware of this problem and did not find it easy to walk into a sitting area and begin conversation. Residents are a captive audience who have become used to receiving whoever wishes to walk in. I felt that it would be difficult for them to find a way of showing me that they did not wish for my company. For example, I might go into a sitting area, chat to one person and find other people putting down the books they had been reading. Would they rather have been left in quiet? These feelings are echoed by a resident, Mrs Richardson, who said in interview: 'I don't go and visit in other lounges. I don't know whether they appreciate me coming or not. So I stopped visiting, though I have visited about three times.' And it was echoed also by a health visitor, replying to a question about visiting residents. 'It's a chore, embarrassed about whether or not to chat to other residents' she wrote.

My solution was to make a point of asking whether it was all right to sit down and then weigh up whether I was in the way or not. I found that I went more to the four sitting areas which were on corridors (1, 2, 3 and 5, Figures 6.1 and 2) because it was easier to walk past if people were sleeping or busy. The day before I left the home I heard from a senior staff member that the residents in sitting area 4 had been complaining that they never saw me, and had been aware that I went more often to other areas. I explained the dilemma to them and that others had more often invited me to stop and talk. However, the issue of being available without imposing and without reinforcing the dependent role of the resident is real.

In addition to uncertainty about boundaries, another aspect of public living is sharing in one's life. Goffman (1961) gives examples of this from a range of establishments, and I recorded several forms at The Pines.

Residents might feel that other people were listening to all that was going on. Mrs Loosely was talking to me in the sitting room. Several times she said 'You see, there's no privacy' and followed that later with 'They're talking about us'. Yet she did not want to move into the bedroom for the pattern of using the sitting room was so firmly established. I did not know whether the two people talking at the far end of the room had been talking about us or not. Mrs Loosely's hearing was very good and she may well have been right. A few days later as I talked with her she asked: 'Are they talking about us? That's the trouble here – all your business is known.'

There was no doubt that all your business was known. Most of it was transacted in front of other people, and the rest they would hear commented upon. Miss Carrow had had a fall and broken her arm. She was feeling bemused one day when she had a letter from a relative which recounted an incident on holiday. Miss Carrow got this incident out of its real perspective and worried about it for much of the day. Miss Carpenter and Mrs Sidney watched her from the other end of the room. 'There you are you see. She's picked up that letter again. Watch her, look. There, holding it again.'

While there may be much that people are willing to share, there are episodes that they want to keep private. Goffman points out how the normal pattern is to move out from home, to work, to yet another base for leisure or club activities. With each move parts can be left behind that one does not want to share in the new situation. Residential living exposes the individual in all areas. In particular the indignities suffered by residents are witnessed by others. 'You should have gone before lunch' said a staff member to a resident as he went to the lavatory during the meal. Everybody around him would see him slightly demeaned.

Indignities, of course, were by no means always staff-induced. Residents' own silly or stubborn behaviour would also be made public. Even more worrying for them was when they began to lose control over their bodies. Mr Gasden went through a spell when he was wet every evening. Fortunately a staff member realised that he was embarrassed about moving while other people were up because they would see his wet trousers – and she let him stay up until after the others had gone to bed. Mr Jepson was not so lucky. He was wet in the middle of lunch, was told to go off and change, and came back after the others had finished their meal and sat and cried. On another day Mr Fothergill had soiled his trousers. He offered one of the care assistants 50 pence if she would keep quiet about it.

So it is rather more than others knowing one's interests. They know intimate details about one's physical and emotional state. It may be hard to remember that such information ought to be used with utmost discretion. Staff at The Pines sometimes seemed to have forgotten this. They would talk to staff about residents in the hearing of other residents. At its most extreme this would mean comments such as 'He's an evil old person' and, worse, 'Mr McNab has just made a mess upstairs and trodden in it – it's like looking after pigs'. A final example results more from thoughtlessness – a domestic assistant knew that Mr Peters had once cut his wrists in a suicide attempt. Seeing his room-mate's razor around, she said, with residents listening: 'Don't leave Mr Peat's razor lying around; you never know what Mr Peters might do.'

Indiscretion may result from lack of awareness or frustration or tiredness. Staff, on becoming exasperated with a resident, sometimes told other residents about it. A general comment in front of a group of residents was made by a staff member about a resident who was not going to be given a drink because on an earlier occasion she had not finished her drink: 'She's naughty with it, she doesn't half play up.' A few moments later, on meeting another resident, the staff member said to her 'That Mrs Hughes is playing up again'.

Such indiscretion may result from lack of awareness of the effect of one's actions or an inability to sense what others are feeling. In other words, it may not be deliberate harshness or insensitivity. The implication for staff training is that ways must be found to help staff realise the significance of seemingly small events to a resident.

Finally, public living means it is difficult to take life at one's own pace. It is not easy to make a quiet start to the day when bombarded with hearty greetings.

## Effects of public living

Another aspect of public living is that events are conspicuous to all. Mrs Smith had a doctor to visit her one day. The doctor had to walk past another sitting room before reaching her room. In the sitting room that he passed a conversation began amongst residents about how often their own doctor visited. There was no doubt that being visited by a doctor conferred some status and therefore when Mrs Richardson said 'My doctor visits once a month whether I ask for him or not' others became uneasy.

Having visitors seemed to confer status also. Thus Mrs Williams would spend time talking about going out to friends and about the people who were calling to see her that day and the next day. There was enough of a pattern about this and similar events to suggest that she and others needed to build up a picture of life outside the home to impress residents.

The more public the style of living, the more the picture of self-worth seems dependent on ways of maintaining status. There were other ways in which this occurred. A common one was to tell off other residents: 'Don't interrupt, Miss Hacket' said Mrs Sidney in the sitting room. When the drinks trolley was taken round a resident would sometimes ask another 'What will you have?' to be met by the rejoinder 'I shall wait till I'm asked'.

The bad table manners of others have already been mentioned. While it was apparent why some habits were objectionable, there were other situations where the speaker seemed anxious to establish her own position, rather than to comment on the other person. Mr Fothergill described how some people ate from their knives instead of their forks and made it clear that he was used to being with a different sort of person. There were other occasions when he felt the need to establish himself as a worthwhile person. Then he talked about the standing of people he had known in a local town and the respect in which he had been held.

Some residents similarly made comments about others to establish their own position. Miss Carpenter at the table said to Miss Black, who was anxious as to whether her meal had been forgotten, 'Just wait, be patient'. And later, 'Just wait dear, she'll come to you. Oh, some people!' This seemed primarily a way of indicating her own patience and good behaviour.

Thus a part of the explanation for residents' behaviour is the maintenance of self-worth. Another aspect concerns expectations. Tobin and Lieberman's (1976) idea of 'anticipatory institutionalisation' has already been mentioned. They suggest that *in anticipation* of a move to a residential home old people change their picture of themselves, their roles and their capacities. This process is continued within the home when people have to 'manage' the state of being a resident. So people do not just exist and behave without considering their surroundings. They present themselves in ways that they think appropriate, in the same way as people do in any other situation. This is why I tried to find out what picture was held of a good resident.

I asked residents for their own interpretation and the view they thought was held by the staff. They failed to make this distinction and only half of the respondents answered this question. Most people thought 'tolerance' important and most of those characteristics mentioned were passive – 'falling in with everything', 'agreeing with most things', 'contented'. A few answers picked on attributes that were more active – 'being happy', 'being lively', 'being sociable' and 'trying to help'. One person commented that staff expect a resident to join in with things, and 'to be taken out of yourself'.

By contrast the 'bad' resident was described as 'ungrateful', 'miserable', 'moaner', 'disagreeable'; other points mentioned were people who 'chatted about others', and those 'who were inclined to be quarrelsome'. Some of the uncertainties as to the purpose of residential living are contained here. Should residents be expected to be sociable, to join in and even to show gratitude? In spite of uncertainty residents have developed an idea of how they ought to behave, and have started this construction before admission.


THE GAINS AND LOSSES OF RESIDENTIAL LIVING

So far in this chapter there has been an attempt to illustrate the style of living in an old age home by considering procedures (for example, in getting people up or providing meals) and by considering the public aspect of residential living. The constraints and the problems outlined are real and many of them are remediable. It is important at this stage to repeat an earlier statement that the constraints of residential living must not blind us to the constraints of other life-styles. Before admission many residents found their lives restricted and burdened. Entry to a residential home may be preferable to earlier living.

A brochure produced by the local authority (Somerset County Council, 1975) lists some of the pros and cons:

Obviously, when you are living with a large group of people – say 36 or 50 residents in all – it is difficult to provide a truly homely atmosphere. Nevertheless, every effort is made to encourage residents to create their own private living-space and their own individual way of life and staff are very aware of the importance of these needs. In our newer homes most of the residents have a room of their own – this helps.

WHAT DO I GAIN, WHAT DO I LOSE?

You gain by not having to worry about such things as: heating, lighting and cooking arrangements – repairs and replacements to property and furniture – how to get help quickly when you need it.

You have the ready-made companionship of the other residents and a large number of people from which to choose your friends. Skilled care is available at all times, night and day, and the building has been designed or adapted to meet the special needs of elderly people.

Inevitably, there are some disadvantages and there are some sacrifices to be made.

As in any community some loss of privacy is involved and a few restrictions are necessary. Almost certainly you will not be able to take with you all your personal possessions. The Head of the Home however helps people to decide what personal belongings can be accommodated. It is not usually possible for large items of furniture to be brought, but such things as pictures, photographs, ornaments, dressing table sets and even fireside chairs, desks and occasional tables can be and frequently are fitted in. More and more residents are arranging to have their rooms close carpeted and to have one or more of the walls of their room papered.

You will also need to adjust to a routine that the staff will make as flexible as possible, but may not be the one you would choose for yourself.

If you are sharing a room there is a need to consider other people in such things as playing the transistor radio and coming in late at night. Residents are, however, free to come and go as they please and are in fact encouraged to have a life outside of the Home. There are no curfews in our establishments. All the staff ask is that if you plan to be away for a meal or a night you should tell them, as otherwise they will worry about you and start searching for you.

It is also necessary that all drugs and medicines are handed to the Matron for safe-keeping. As certain drugs are dangerous if taken after alcohol, it is wise, in your own interest, to inform the Matron if you are accustomed to taking alcoholic drinks.

It is very important that NO SMOKING takes place in bedrooms as it is far too dangerous and places are set aside in the Home for smoking.

Our staff are aware of the snags and of the problems faced by the residents and they do try very hard to help and give a personal service.

Only you can judge if this kind of life is the best that is available to you. We believe that for a great many it is the best answer.

Most residents at The Pines thought they had made the right decision and twenty-two out of twenty-three respondents stressed that they would advise a friend to live in a residential home. There were three or four provisos to this – 'If there was nothing else to do' said one person, 'if you couldn't do the work' said another, while a third said 'if you had nobody to rely on'. The reasons for this nearly all fell into the areas covered by one of the paragraphs from the brochure. 'You gain by not having to worry about such things as: heating, lighting and cooking arrangements – repairs and replacements to property and furniture – how to get help quickly when you need it.'

Mrs Richardson expressed this clearly. 'The most important thing was feeling comfortable – nothing to worry about. I was able to rest, I'd done my duty. I was surprised at such a place.'

Residents were glad to have people to do things for them – washing, ironing, helping with getting to bed, bathing, dressing, doing errands. The other area that was mentioned by several people was that of having staff around. 'To have someone around', 'someone able to give you attention', 'somebody there when you're ill', 'bells' (to ring if assistance was needed) were some of the points mentioned.

When asked what they enjoyed most about living in a residential home most answers were to do with 'comfort', 'peacefulness', 'rest' and the provision of services. The kindness of staff was mentioned: 'nothing is too much trouble'.

A similar question was asked by Peace *et al.* (1979). They found that residents, when asked the one thing they liked best about living in the home, stated: a room of one's own (24 replies), material comforts (20), the care and attention (20), being looked after (20), the staff (11), the 'home from home' atmosphere (9), matron (5).

It is significant that activities were not mentioned in this list and at The Pines, where residents were not limited to one answer, only Miss Carpenter stressed activities as the most enjoyable factor. She said that she enjoyed the TV, entertainments, Christmas ('I enjoyed that very much indeed'), birthdays ('they all sing to you'). While others mentioned activities such as watching slide shows as enjoyable, nobody else stated activities were the best part of residential living. It would seem that such a life-style is regarded as freeing *from* burdens rather than freeing *to* do other things.

This is probably significant in relation to companionship and friendship. The fact has been mentioned that many residents stated the importance of having people around to help. This provides freedom *from* anxiety about what would happen if they fell and were alone, or were ill. Only Mrs Tanner mentioned company as one of the positives and she found a childhood friend in the home. Most stated that they did not have a special friend and this is similar to Townsend's (1962) findings.

These examples suggest how important it is to distinguish between social isolation and loneliness in old age. People who were unmarried and had led an isolated life tended not to complain about loneliness unless they had lost contact with a close friend. Those who had lost or been separated from someone they loved often felt lonely even when they had lived with other people. In fact the majority seemed to feel their loss more keenly, because there were fewer opportunities of losing themselves in household activities and relationships with other members of their families and friends.

People who are separated from past significant relationships (particularly spouse or children) do not expect to replace those by new deep relationships. However, companionship may help to make other losses bearable. In talking about friendship residents were clear that they had no special friends. One resident stated that she did not like to pick out one person for attention, another that she never had had special friends. However, the style of public living may lead people to question the attitudes of others towards them. For example, Mrs Knight said: 'None are close friends, they are acquaintainces. It's hard to tell who your friends are. I hear quickly – and hear a lot of things I'm not meant to.' (She did add that she felt the same uncertainty outside.)

Mrs Draxton said that there was one person she thought she had made friends with but now she was not so sure. Living from a public base – the sitting area – means that others are seen over long periods, not just when one chooses and this fact, together with the jealousy that occurs when residents observe the activities of others, seems to discourage the forming of close relationships. Townsend (1962) found that 'fewer friendships were formed between persons sleeping in one room than between persons sleeping in single rooms'. Privacy may increase the likelihood of relationships being formed.

It is also important to note that only one person stated she was lonely 'quite often'. Most claimed they were never lonely and here there was frequent mention of other people: 'never lonely – there are always people around'; 'not at all lonely – so many people'; 'I'm lonely when I'm depressed, but there are people around'. The presence of other people reduced loneliness.

Two residents mentioned that the other residents were not the sort of people they would have chosen to live with, and it should be noted that residents had virtually no choice of where they sat in the dining hall or in sitting rooms. There were few situations where one might meet residents other than those from one's table or sitting area. Bingo was one of the few events where this happened.

The aspect of living with other residents that was disliked most was bad manners. However, some people who 'poked their noses in', were 'too religious', or 'too filthy in their talk' caused offence as well. Most stated they were not concerned about confused residents – 'you feel sorry for them' – though one or two incidents of wandering or finding a strange person in one's bed had been frightening. There was little problem about losing possessions, though one man recounted sharing a bedroom with a man who

didn't know what was his and someone else's. It can be very uncomfortable like that. You just make sure you don't lose too much. One chap I think had been a professional burglar! Still staff will get things back. He used to get up at three in the morning and I'd think, 'Now what's he up to ?'.

Inevitably some people found it difficult to live with others; on such occasions staff might move one of the residents. In the meantime the tension was considerable and Mrs Williams described how one resident had taken everything out of her hands. 'She was the same at the table in the beginning. "You don't want to do that. There's attendants to do that." One day I nearly ran away – it was all too much.'

One factor that surprised the residents was that there were few restrictions. They were pleased to have visitors when they wanted and the more active would go out for a walk or shopping without having to tell staff where they were going.

## TASKS IN RESIDENTIAL LIVING

Townsend (1972) distinguishes three systems of occupation for inmates. 'Two are formally organised in institutions by the management. These are maintenance work of various kinds and occupational instruction or "therapy".' The third system is personal services among inmates.

## (1)  *Maintenance work*
This phrase is used to indicate work that is essential to the basic running of the establishment. Half-a-dozen residents would sometimes help with drying up, usually two after each meal. These residents would finish their meal and then dry up the few items that had not been finished. There were times when the request for help from staff was met grudgingly. A senior staff member asked Miss Carpenter to help dry up. 'Oh, my arthritis, I don't know' was the reply. Later Miss Carpenter said to two other residents: 'She asked me to dry up but I can't because of my legs.' Later still she was drying up. Usually residents were glad to help. It was a sign of their greater ability and it allowed them into a domain (the kitchen) that was exclusive to staff on most occasions; it allowed them also to meet residents from different sitting rooms and tables. Mrs Williams dried up and listened to the staff conversation. She smiled and said to me: 'I have lots of laughter just noticing what goes on.'

I was surprised that residents did nothing to clear the tables. In fact the reason probably was that staff cleared items away so promptly that there was little for the residents to do.

Miss Johns was the only resident who made a significant contribution to the running of the home. She laid up the tables for lunch and tea; often collected the cups after drinks had been taken round and washed them up. She was younger than most other residents, only 67, and had been transferred from the old workhouse. The care assistants were grateful for her help and gave her a special Christmas present.

Other help was only slight. Some residents made their beds, a few did some dusting. Mrs Richardson occasionally buttered some bread for tea. Mrs Quigley saw something was spilt in the sitting area and went to get a brush and dustpan – which was most unusual. Involvement in any tasks to do with running the establishment was slight. A few residents did a little. There is, of course, no clear picture as to the demands that ought to be made on residents. However, Tunstall (1966) showed that with his sample housework was the activity that provided the second most pleasure. Consequently there may be a link between the purposelessness felt by some residents and the minimal involvement (non-existent for most residents) in the running of the establishment. It is significant also that residents probably had more time available and less that they *needed* to do than at any other time in their adult lives.

## (2)  *Occupational instruction*
There were two occasions when someone came to teach the residents how to make Christmas decorations. These were the only examples of

occupational instruction because the home had not got the services of
an occupational therapist.

(3)  *Personal services among inmates*

Initially I was struck by the passivity of residents and the little amount
of help they gave to one another. In fact more thorough investigation
showed a much larger system of helping than had been imagined. At
meals some residents would collect the sticks and zimmer frames of
others and place them out of the way. Miss Tippitt wiped the chairs
and helped two residents who sat at her table. Mrs Quigley agreed to
mend a dress for Mrs Sidney. She asked Miss Hacket to collect it from
the bedroom since Miss Hacket shared with Mrs Sidney. Mrs Quigley
then mended it. A staff member, incidentally, said: 'You needn't have
bothered to do that. We'd have done it for her.' Some more able people
were willing to get things for others. Mrs Pinker was blind and Mrs
Smith would read the paper to her and help when she got stuck with
her knitting. Mrs Richardson put a hot water bottle on the chair of a
day visitor each day to warm it up for her. It was common for one
resident to attract the attention of a staff member for another; similarly they would remind each other that it was time for tea, or time to
come out of the bedroom to collect a drink. At night-time if they heard
someone fall they might ring their alarm bell to attract the staff.

However, there was a clear understanding that residents should not
help each other with moving about. Residents stated the reason was the
staff fear that both helper and helped might fall, so making the situation worse. Mrs Williams was one of several who said how hard it was
to see other people struggle and to do nothing. In fact she said one
day that she had been helping the sick, 'though I know I'm not meant
to'. On another occasion Mrs Quigley helped Mrs White stand up to
go off to the toilet. She explained what she had done to a care assistant.
'I just helped her up. She has walked along to the toilet and she'll call
you when she needs you.'

Townsend (1972) found that the infirm were less likely to help others
and this was the case also at The Pines, though some of the more able
performed no services for others.

### PROVISION OF FACILITIES

Staff in a residential home have to decide how many facilities to provide on the premises. Cost may be one factor to consider but the more
difficult one is whether residents should be encouraged to look outside
the home for their needs.

At The Pines a small stock of goods was kept and taken round to
residents about twice a week. The stock included sweets, cigarettes and
toiletries. Mrs Quigley and Miss Carpenter started just before I left to

ake the trolley-load of goods round the home; until then it had been
aken by a staff member. How well stocked should such a 'shop' be?

A hairdresser came regularly once or twice a week and residents
were very grateful for the service, which boosted their self-image.

Posting letters was more difficult, since there was no postbox on the
premises. Mrs Richardson would leave her letters prominently on the
coffee table and wait for a staff member to ask 'Does this need posting?'.
She would need to check up to ensure that the letter really had been
posted. In fact a postbox would have made her less dependent on staff,
for she could have posted the letters in an internal box herself and been
more confident that they would not be forgotten, since it would have
been emptied by the postman. So perhaps the difficult question should
be tackled by the extent to which provision of facilities increases the
independence of residents.

Mrs Roberts wished there was a phone in a place that was comfortable and private. Residents were dependent for incoming calls on staff
passing on messages or staff calling them to the phone in the office to
receive a call and were unable to phone anybody themselves unless in
exceptional circumstances they asked to use the office phone. Staff were
often willing to make arrangements for residents – they phoned for a
taxi for Mrs Richardson – but residents remained unnecessarily dependent.

Indeed, an additional indicator of residential life, and one not used
in this study, is *accessibility to the outside world*. This would document
procedures for visitors (notices, arrangements, hours, privacy) and the
residents' access to the outside (arrangements for posting and receiving
letters, use of phone, spending time outside the home). This indicator
might provide some clues to staff attitudes to residents. Accessibility to
the world outside a residential establishment is significant in most institutions. Relatives and patients are concerned about times and conditions for hospital visiting. Anxiety about the posting of letters had been
an important factor in the lead-up to riots at two boys' approved schools
(HMSO, 1947, 1959). There were differences (censorship was not an
issue in an old people's home) but the uncertainty about whether mail
had been forgotten was similar.

What views are held by staff and others of the appropriate life-style
for the elderly? Should residents be restricted like prisoners or as free
as hotel guests? Should messages for residents be given to staff to be
passed on to residents, as happens with most communications from
official bodies?

## A RESIDENT'S DAY

Mrs Richardson talked about life at The Pines and later wrote some
notes about three days. She emerges as someone who is less active than

some (she could only get around on crutches) but who is contented. This fuller picture of life for one resident concludes this chapter.

Nothing is boring. After lunch I come in my room and read my Bible for an hour. After tea I come in between six and seven and read the Bible again. Don't read anything else, got no time. Still sometimes mend and sew. I write letters – two or three letters – spend about three-quarters of an hour writing. About three o'clock I sleep for ten minutes. Not interested in TV. Put up with it and say nothing. Don't want them to feel 'she's up against it'. I look forward to meals to move about – not really hungry, could do without dinner – we're not really doing anything. I do butter the bread and help do some sprouts, that depends who's on. Like to feel I'm doing something.

It's mortal cold so it's easier to sit still than get up and walk around. I don't go and visit in other lounges. Do they appreciate me coming or not? So I stopped visiting though I have visited about three times. From our sitting room everyone goes to bed at eight-thirty. I have some tablets to help me go to sleep. I sleep and wake up about two or three. My leg hurts, feel it's a long time. Have some visitors, two or three one week, none the next. Still go to meetings (religious groups) in my brother's home, have done right from a girl. Religion is what makes me happy.

Mrs Richardson also wrote some notes about what she felt on three particular days.

*Thursday:* It's now 1.10 and I have just come back from dinner, steak and kidney pie, cabbage, potatoes, ice-cream and peaches. I was asked if I would butter some bread for tea so 3.30 I go and do it and come back again 3.55. The butter was nice and soft and made it easy. When 5 o'clock came it was tea-time so here we go again for tea. We had cold meat and chips, quite nice, and cake to finish. At 7 o'clock I go to my room and spend a quiet time alone yet not alone with my Bible. I come back again and at 8.30 go off to bed, take a sleeping tablet and when I do go to sleep I dream, some not very nice, I can't seem to get through the jobs and it worries me.

*Friday:* And here goes again. The lady that sits with me each day comes in for the day and has dinner and tea; so every Tuesday and Friday she sees the nurse, so in comes the nurse to give her a liver injection and back she comes again. Mr X wasn't down for breakfast and dinner so his chair was empty for breakfast and at dinner-time a Mr Y took the chair. He is a very nice man, he filled our glasses with water. He has a long walk, he comes for dinner and goes again and comes back for tea. His wife is in a home, her mind is in a bad state, he really has lots to do by the time he visits his wife and cares for the home. Most Fridays we have fish for dinner but today we had bacon and eggs for dinner and cabbage and potatoes but *we do like* the nice piece of fish fried in deep fat and some potatoes.

For tea we had a meat and egg pie, it was nice. After we had tea we came back to our room and one lady came in to say there is a man in our toilet with the door wide open. I said call the attendant and down she comes. She said: 'What are you doing in the ladies' toilet? Make haste and get out of it.' He said: 'I am sorry.' He so often does this and says the same. I have at 7 a cup of coffee and then at 8.30 off to bed.

*Saturday:* It is now 10.45 and a poor man of 97 tried to walk down and when he got to my seat he could not go any further, so done up. And the lady that comes in every day doesn't come in Saturdays or Sundays so he was able to sit beside me and then the attendant came and took him back in a wheelchair.

We had nice fried fish for our dinner today. I have a taxi man to take me to Moorhinch once a fortnight so I asked Matron to phone for Sunday a.m. and she has tried all day so now tonight at 7 she at last got through and I have just worried most of the day. You see he is cheap so I want to have him if I can.

Now I have just had my orange drink and 8.30 will soon be here and then off to bed. I go out early on Sunday morning at 9.45.

# Chapter 7

———◆———

## MR JEPSON and MRS WILLIAMS –
## PICTURES OF TWO RESIDENTS

After I had completed my stay at The Pines I decided it would be useful to gather together my research notes on some residents. I selected two whom I had known well and whose personalities and responses to residential living were very different. Had I made this decision earlier the notes would have been fuller but all my interaction would have been changed.

The bulk of the material comes from brief research notes; there are shorter sections from interviews, life satisfaction tests and questionnaires completed by relatives.

### MR JEPSON

*October*

There was a gruff mutter from the end of the corridor. When it was repeated I heard 'Open the door then'. Mr Jepson was standing outside the lavatory door on his zimmer frame and couldn't open it. I felt a bit annoyed at the brusqueness of his demand.

One lunch he pushed back his chair at the end of the meal and knocked into someone else. 'You'll have to be more careful' said one of the staff. Comments all round – one woman muttered about it, another said to me 'You have to take no notice of them, that's what I do'. The care assistant added 'They're just like children'.

While I was sitting chatting with him in his sitting area he gave me an apple. Later, when he saw a new resident being pushed past in a wheelchair, 'She's an awkward one, always being awkward' he stated.

One night I was calling numbers for bingo. Mr Jepson was playing and I heard him being told off by another resident, Mr Fothergill, for offering money (1p) for a stake to one of the women. 'You're embarrassing her' said the man. Mr Jepson was deflated and the row fizzled down.

Later that night he was one of a few residents still up watching TV after 9 o'clock. That was his regular practice, staff said.

He came out of the lift to go into breakfast and looked at the slow-moving procession of people on zimmer frames and with sticks in front of him. 'To come to this, it's strange how it happens, you're all right one day' he muttered.

At lunch he got up to go to the lavatory. He refused the offer of a wheelchair. After lunch he emerged – he had wet himself. A care assistant took him up to change him and he came back to finish his lunch. Then he sat and cried. A care assistant put her arm round him. 'It's all right' she said. A resident and cleaner nodded their heads in sympathy for him.

*November*
After chatting in the sitting area, he got up and on to his zimmer, he was very shaky and angry with a resident who was in his way. I thought that was because he was frightened of falling. 'Awful to be like this, awful', as he slowly went off. Later at lunch he was helped on to his chair by another resident.

*December*
He gave some sweets to a care assistant.

*January*
I was in a sitting area chatting to residents. A care assistant came in. 'Mr Jepson's being awful, he keeps ringing the bell – he wants his zip undone, wants his trousers down, wants his trousers up. Oh, I told him he'd get a kick up the arse if he didn't get on.' Other residents commented: 'You can't be on all the time'; 'He's getting worse, wants more and more done for him'. The care assistant: 'He says he can't walk now. Staff laugh at the way I talk to him but I can't be on all the time. Yesterday I kept my hand over the buzzer and he pulled his own trousers up.'

Later in his sitting area he joined in a discussion about prices. Then after offering me a sherry he talked about sudden changes in health and how awful it was.

The next day he was sitting in a downstairs room (he'd been put there because it wasn't so far for him to get to meals). Another resident was trying to cheer him up. 'I can't understand what's happened to me. Life isn't worth living. I was in the church for forty-four years but I don't believe in Jesus – he's not authentic. Why is there all this suffering? I must have been very bad.' A staff member came by and stroked his bald head. He looked round and smiled at her. Then he asked me to get a wheelchair to get him to the toilet quickly. I got him there in time.

He was sitting upstairs again the next day and rang the bell. When I went up he wanted a chair in which to go down to lunch. 'Should I take him down?' I asked the senior staff member, aware of the policy of getting him to walk. She came up and eventually there was a compromise. I helped him to get downstairs and then he had a wheelchair from the lift into the dining room. He had to go to the lavatory before he set off downstairs and again as soon as he got down. 'It's these water tablets [diuretics]' he commented.

After lunch a few days later I took him to the toilet and then to the lift in the wheelchair. He had to walk from there. I got him on to his zimmer and then he couldn't move. Others were standing round waiting to use the lift. I tried to direct the traffic, Mr Jepson fell; I put him in a wheelchair and got him back to his sitting room. He seemed all right.

He was back in the downstairs sitting room. He called me and wanted to know how I would write the report. How would I put in people's opinions when there's disagreement, say, about getting people to walk. I explained that I should put in both sides. Two care assistants came up: 'You told your son all about us last night, then.' A discussion followed, and it became clear that he had talked about being made to walk. 'We have to do what the doctor says, what Matron says, what's for your good' said one. 'You have to understand why we are doing it' said the other.

At lunch I started to push his chair up to the table. 'Bob [a resident] says I have to do it myself' he said. At the end of the meal a care assistant said: 'You go to the toilet now and you won't need a wheelchair.' I went off to the bank. Half an hour later I was back and Mr Jepson was coming back from the toilet. Two staff were talking about him. 'He had a bottle just near him and he's done it all over his trousers and shoes.' I didn't know whether he heard or not, but he stood still with his jaw set. 'I'm in hot water now' he said to me.

Then he was told to go upstairs and change. He became the focus of attention, with several staff round alternately encouraging, bantering, ignoring him.

'That other care assistant would get the chair for me' he had said. 'I don't want it all the time, just when I want to do a wee quickly.' There was a discussion about whether that was good for Mr Jepson or not. 'She'd wheel you all everywhere. Anyway she'll be back tomorrow.'

Someone else came by. 'New shoes, Mr Jepson?' 'No', said a care assistant, 'they're wet'. 'No they're not', replied Mr Jepson, and showed me his trousers (which were wet) to prove they were dry. 'Life isn't worth living' he had muttered earlier.

*February*
Upstairs Mr Fothergill talked about Mr Jepson. 'He's not like his brother, this one is dirty with bad manners; it only makes it worse if you talk to him.' Mr Jepson was standing nearby.

Later when trying to walk downstairs he kept saying he was stuck.

'Are there any tissues down here?' he asked a care assistant. 'Have you got some upstairs?' she replied. 'Yes, but I've not been up' said Mr Jepson. 'I'll bring some down when I come' she promised.

'Time to go to the toilet' he muttered. 'Oh I can't get up . . . it's these tablets.'

He was joking with different staff and other residents. He seemed more prepared to laugh at himself about getting up and sitting down. When he fell back into his chair I tried to help him. 'No, I've got to do it' he said.

That afternoon there was a lively conversation going on in the sitting room. They talked about their past lives, places they had all known. 'I caught the train and walked to the end of the lane. Buffalo Bill was here then', Mr Jepson joined in. (He often talked about Buffalo Bill and I was never sure to what he was referring.) 'Are you all right?' he asked someone who was whimpering with a headache. Then he talked about playing bingo and going out to the Red Cross club.

One of the staff told me about Mr Jepson's worry about his dog, Scamp, and whether it had been put down or not. 'It would break your heart to leave a pet behind' she added.

At breakfast he had been moved to a different table and he was chatting and laughing more than I had ever heard him. He would not sit in the sitting room in the chair of someone who had just died. 'He is the only one I've ever known make a fuss' said a staff member.

The next day at lunch he pushed his plate away halfway through the meal and resisted all attempts to get him to eat.

He complained to me about the effect of the tablets he was taking. 'It's not worth having them if they make you feel so rotten, I'd rather die.' After lunch he was again complaining about them, in a strange muddled conversation that I couldn't follow about going to the toilet at four and about going down the drain.

Two care assistants talked about him while having their lunch – one of them had taken him to the toilet in a wheelchair. Would another care assistant object? 'She does go on about it' was the reply. 'They're human after all. I had to leave the room this morning because I couldn't stand hearing Mrs Jones [care assistant] going on at Mr Jepson. It's awful to see him crying.'

A senior staff member talked about the possibility of getting Mr Jepson assessed at a geriatric hospital.

A group of staff were around when Mr Jepson came back to the sitting area. They were anxious to see him settled and had made him a special bag to hang from his zimmer frame to hold some of his possessions. 'Come on Ben', said someone, 'you must stand', as he was being moved from the wheelchair to his armchair. 'That's better, you can do it as well as I.' They looked around. 'Where is his this?' 'Where is his that?' they asked each other, but not him.

He was dozing when I walked past at 10.20 a.m. A few minutes later, in another sitting area, the staff came round with a trolley and morning drinks. They talked about Mr Jepson who had sworn at one of them at breakfast. 'It's getting him up in the morning' said one care assistant. 'I made him apologise' said the other. 'Well, it's a pity he swears' added a resident.

I heard Mr Jepson calling out. He wanted to go to the toilet. Someone helped me get him in to a wheelchair. He talked about his tablets being changed (though he was a bit muddled) and wanted to know if I would be around at lunch-time.

When I brought him back from the toilet a group of staff stood round Mr Jepson. He was talking about how he'd rather be a woman. 'They get treated differently' he said. 'He'd rather you helped him today than me' said the care assistant at whom he'd sworn.

Before lunch two care assistants tried to help him walk to the toilet, a distance of only 10 yards. 'You've got to walk – you've got half an hour to get into the toilet and back – doctor's orders – got to go – stand up straight – you're not going to sit down – now you're stood up – go on – one, two, that's a good boy – quiet now, Mr Jepson [she's shouting! ] – don't ring that bell, one, two, one, two – look where you're going or you'll fall – concentrate on what you're doing.' It took him nearly half an hour, full of stops and starts, cajoling, threatening. Lunch seemed very quiet – I wondered if residents had been affected by seeing his struggle.

During the staff lunch care assistants talked about Mr Jepson. 'He keeps ringing the bell when he's in bed. He says pass the bottle when he can reach it, then he rings to put the bottle back, then rings for something else. One of the staff takes his bell away. It's much harder getting people up in the mornings now. So many need help. Mr Jepson is the biggest problem.' She recounts how at breakfast Mr Jepson had said when he saw her: 'Look who's here then, oh goodness, f—— me', to which she had replied 'Don't you swear at me'. 'I was flabbergasted' she added. They discussed how much easier it would be for staff to take residents in wheelchairs than to make them walk.

Later another care assistant said she thought he was frightened of two of the care assistants. 'He gets worried at them shouting at him, that's why he's worse today.'

That afternoon two care assistants were standing laughing. In spite of the fact that they were laughing at me, he was convinced that they were laughing at him, as he came back from the toilet. He talked about it a lot, saying to me 'They shouldn't giggle at me', and later stopped another care assistant to say 'Jill, I was coming down the corridor and they were laughing at me'.

When the drinks were taken round one care assistant said to another 'You're getting a better reception from Mr Jepson than I did'. 'I can't help it if I'm sympathetic to him' was the reply.

I took him to the toilet during lunch and he squeezed my hand afterwards.

I sat talking in his sitting area. Another resident would interrupt every now and again with 'Say "thank you" ' or 'What do you say?' as I passed him his cup of tea or helped him with something. Mr Jepson talked about his time in the army, playing football for the army XI when he'd played at half-back. He had driven a truck across Luxembourg to play a match and got back to base early the next morning. Then he told me about friends he used to have in Cornwall and a nurse whom he'd met recently in hospital. She had given him a tie, and he'd promised to be the best man at her wedding, 'but I won't get there now'.

*March*

Mr Jepson had been taken off all tablets. He was not walking at all and was to go for day care and assessment.

I took him to the toilet. He wanted to sit there and chat – I left him and came back later.

After lunch he went to the toilet. He came back very pleased: 'I have done my job.'

I sat in his sitting room and he was one of a group that talked about rugby and a recent international.

Before lunch I sat in his sitting area and he talked about life and death and his time in the home. 'You're finished and not finished' he said. He meant that life was not worth living, he'd got nothing left and no longer believed in anything to come.

In the afternoon one of the care assistants tried to get him interested in looking at a magazine, but did not succeed. Another assistant managed to get him to walk in to meals, unusual because he nearly always had a wheelchair.

He went off to hospital for the day.

He seemed weaker on his legs; he put no weight on his frame to help move from an armchair to the wheelchair. He talked in a muddled way, not knowing where he was; he remembered getting up but then couldn't remember anything.

He again walked back from lunch, persuaded by a particular care assistant. A contrast with the day before when he did not even stand.

I told him about my car which had gone wrong. The ignition switch had not been working and he understood perfectly. Then he asked what his duties were. I talked about retirement, that someone else was doing his job. 'Who's my boss, then? Who pays me?' so I explained that Matron ran the home and that he got a pension.

Later on in the office two staff members talked about him and suggested that going off to hospital each day – a journey of several miles – unsettled him. On Friday he had come back in the ambulance and said: 'Why are you leaving me here? I want to go home.'

Mr Jepson was to be admitted to hospital for a short stay. If they could not improve anything he would return to the home and await the next hospital vacancy.

He talked very knowledgeably to me about football, he recalled his time in Luxembourg and then mentioned a court martial he had taken part in. He said later: 'I am not able to sort things out in part of my brain.'

## April

Mr Jepson returned from hospital. They had not been able to do much and would take him back on a permanent basis when they had a vacancy.

He was sleeping while I talked to other residents. Then he woke up: 'You are taking up a lot of room. How are things?' (I had been away over Easter.)

I heard an assistant shouting 'I told you not to ring that bell', and a staff member commented 'That's Mr Jepson in trouble'.

I shaved him later that day and then we talked about recent league football matches.

He told me how one of the senior staff had said he'd kept her awake all night, 'Old Nick was coming through the door with a knife to get me' he said, and got very angry with another resident who didn't know who Old Nick was. He repeated the story several times. He was worried about keeping people awake but seemed a bit happier when I said that other people got nightmares.

A resident in another sitting area complained about being woken up by Mr Jepson. 'I couldn't get back to sleep.'

A senior staff member said that she had joked with Mr Jepson and pretended that he'd woken her up.

I helped him fill in his postal vote for the local elections. He talked about politics and the local councillors: 'I don't believe in wasting votes. I've got no patience with those who grumble and don't vote.'

*May*

Mr Jepson was admitted to hospital. Staff recounted to me how upset he'd been, crying and asking 'What have I done wrong? Why do I have to go down the union?'

I visited him in hospital the next day and took in some clothes. He was coherent and talked about the ward but constantly returned to his question about why he had to be there. Was it because he had been naughty and been wet? He cried occasionally and asked to see one of the women staff of whom he'd been very fond.

A senior staff member went in to see him. He told her about his feelings for a care assistant at the home and how he would like to see her. He was scared he had done something wrong. 'I told him that we should keep his bed for him. I shouldn't say it, but what can you do?' she said, to me.

I arrived at the home to hear it was Mr Jepson's funeral. He was 87. Three members of staff and a resident had gone. They came back and described it as a very cold affair. 'I wish he could have stayed here' said someone. One of the residents had been in to see him at lunch-time on Tuesday and he had died soon after. A staff member commented how he had accepted the short visit to hospital for assessment but not the permanent stay.

## A RELATIVE'S PERSPECTIVE

Mr Jepson's son, aged between 50 and 60, visited his father for a quarter of an hour every day. He (the son) had decided admission to the home was necessary. 'My wife died some three years previously of cancer and it became impossible for me to keep house for an aged father and myself when his medical condition became so unpredictable.'

He had sometimes felt sad about his father's admission. 'Probably a little self-pity. A very happy family shattered by a mother dying of thrombosis, wife of cancer and father becoming degenerate.' (Probably means 'going downhill' or 'becoming confused').

He thought the best things about the home were the comfort of the furnishings, very good food, the pleasant attitude of all the staff, the opportunity of conversing with your own age-group; the worst things were the inability of all the inmates to live for each other, single bedrooms, the lack of ground-space in which to walk and being pestered by do-gooders at Christmas.

Residents were very well looked after but might profit from being fussed less by staff 'so that the inmates played a more active part in the home'. Old people should 'create a hobby and interest other people' and 'I think it would be good if some form of physical training or suitable exercises could be organised to keep inmates fitter and occupied. Not so much use of drugs but more use of the human being – less drugs – more keep-fit.'

When old he would wish to live in an old people's home 'so as to retain as much independence as possible without having to worry about my degeneration.'

This information is taken from a questionnaire completed by Mr Jepson's son.

## MR JEPSON'S OWN VIEW (interview in February)

Mr Jepson had some knowledge of the home before his admission from visiting friends there. He described the day at his own home when he had been 'reading the Sunday paper and the floor came up to him'. His son had said that something must be done and had seen a doctor at the hospital.

He talked about settling in:

I was used to the army. John and Bob [other residents] told you about things, what was expected . . . I accept discipline as it comes . . . the food is OK. I couldn't bring anything in with me [his interpretation of the policy of the home]. I would like to have brought my dog. I ask now about Scamp, and Charley [a friend who visits] says 'We let a lady have him' and I'm sure I saw him out in the street once.